Detox Drin Fasting - Detoxification & Fat Burning Smoothies (Best Detox Smoothies & Fasting Diet Juicing Recipes) + Smoothies Are Like You

Smoothie Food Poetry For The Smoothie Lifestyle - Poem A Day Book (Poem For Mom & Smoothie Gift & Smoothie Guide For Beginners in Rhymes, Verses & Quotes For Smoothie Lifestyle Recipe Journal) - 2 In 1 Box Set Compilation

By Juliana Baldec

"Thank you for this wonderful compilation ! I have bought books of your before but this stuns it all. I am very happy with it. Thanks !."-- Liv

Detox Drinks With Juice Fasting Detoxification & Fat Burning Smoothies + Smoothies Are Like You by Juliana Baldec

All rights reserved. No part of this publication may be reproduced or transmitted in any form or by any means, electronic or mechanical, including photocopy, recording or any information storage and retrieval system, without prior permission in writing from the publisher.

© 2014 by Juliana Baldec

Learn more:

www.facebook.com/healthysmoothiesrecipes

Detox Drinks With Juice Fasting Detoxification & Fat Burning Smoothies + SmoothiesAre Like You by Juliana Baldec

Bonus	7
Book 1: SMOOTHIES: 16 Blender Recipes For Smoothie Diet & Detox Diet	9
Why You Should Read This Book	10
My Favorite Smoothie Quote	21
My Personal Rules For Weight Loss With These Smoothies	22
Smoothie 1: Strawberry N'Creams	23
Smoothie 2: Mango/Papaya Protein Booster	26
Smoothie 3: Superfood Greens Shake	29
Smoothie 4: Exotic Coconut & Green Superpower Ginger Smoothie	32
Smoothie 5: Rich Berry Screamer	36
Smoothie 6: Vanilla Smoothie Delight	39
Smoothie 7: Purple Power Booster	43
Smoothie 8: Kefir Peanut Butter Breakfast Smoothie	46
Smoothie 9: Blueberry Pecan & Vanilla Smoothie	49
Smoothie 10: Avocado Banana Berry Avalanche	53
Smoothie 11: Hazel Banana Vanilla Walnut Cream Smoothie	57
Smoothie 12: The Beta Carotene Energy Booster	60
Smoothie 13: The Blackberry Blueberry Blue Preserve Energy Triangle	63
Smoothie 14: The Coffee'n Cream Cinnamon Smoothie Booster	66
Smoothie 15: The Peanut Butter Banana Silk	69
Smoothie 16: The Golden Delight	72
Interactive Nutritious Ways	75
Blender Recipes For Weight Loss Quiz	78
Notes	79
Answers	80
Conclusion	81

www.facebook.com/healthysmoothierecipes

Book 2 JUICING: Juicing For Vitality 85

My Favorite Quote 86

Why You Should Read This Book 87

Introduction 91

The 5 Minute 6 Step Juicing System 95

Notes 98

Why My Juicing Diet Works (My Secret Morning Elixir Ritual & Benefits) 99

Strawberry Carrot Beautifier 102

Lime Lemon Jalapeno Ginger Gold 105

Grapefruit Cranberry Double Immune System Blaster 109

Zesty Blackberry Ginger Booster 121

Blueberry Coconut Veggie Detoxer 124

Orange Breakfast Power Cocktail 130

Full Body Detoxer 135

Green Gold Juice 138

Beet & Black Radish Liver Cleanser 144

Exotic Strawberry Rasperry Vitality Drink 147

Notes 150

Juicing For Vitality & Energy The Smart Way 154

Effortless Juicing Process (Juicing Has Never Been Easier) 157

Power Up Your Juicing Habits With Healing & Detoxifiying Wheat Grass Elixirs 160

Green Star Juicer Review 163

Breville Speed Juice Extractor Review 166

Juicing For Vitality Quiz 170

Answers 172

www.facebook.com/healthysmoothiesrecipes

Conclusion	173
More Information	177
Notes	179
More Information	180
Book 3: Smoothies Are Like You	182
Why Smoothie Poems?	184
Dedication	190
Smoothies Are Like A	192
Smoothies Are Like B	194
Smoothies Are Like C	196
Smoothies Are Like D	198
Smoothies Are Like E	200
Smoothies Are Like F	202
Smoothies Are Like G	204
Smoothies Are Like H	206
Smoothies Are Like I	208
Smoothies Are Like J	210
Smoothies Are Like K	212
Smoothies Are Like L	214
Smoothies Are Like M	216
Smoothies Are Like N	218
Smoothies Are Like O	220
Smoothies Are Like P	222
Smoothies Are Like Q	224
Smoothies Are Like R	226
Smoothies Are Like S	228
Smoothies Are Like T	230
Smoothies Are Like U	232

Smoothies Are Like V 234

Smoothies Are Like W 236

Smoothies Are Like X 238

Smoothies Are Like Y 240

Smoothies Are Like Z 242

Conclusion 244

More Scrumptiousness 245

About The Author 246

More Information 248

Bonus

Dear Smoothie lover ...If you'd like to get some more healthy & delicious smoothie recipes that you can add to your daily meal plan as you follow along with these healthy smoothie for weight loss recipes, you can download it for free for a very limited time by going here:

http://www.facebook.com/healthysmoothiesrecipes

Enjoy!

Juliana Baldec

www.facebook.com/healthysmoothiesrecipes

Book 1: SMOOTHIES: 16 Blender Recipes For Smoothie Diet & Detox Diet

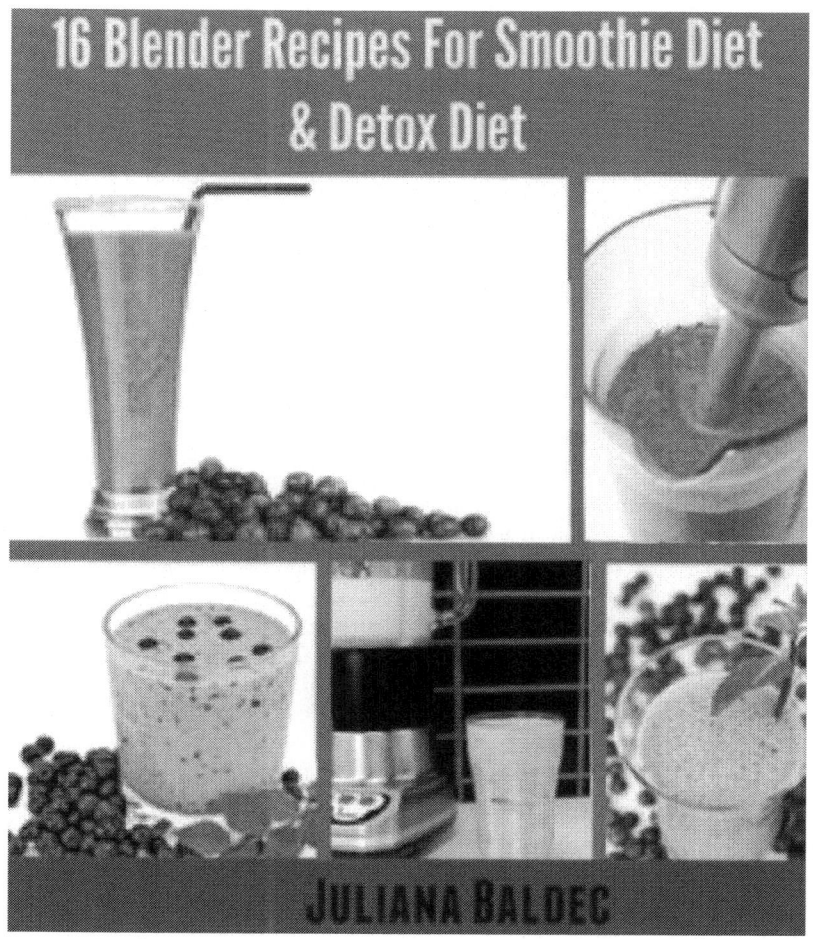

www.facebook.com/healthysmoothierecipes

Why You Should Read This Book

You should read this book because in this book you will find superfoods that are very beneficial for your health and they will keep your body lean and clean.

Taking in all these superfoods via smoothies on a daily basis is going to benefit you because you are going to keep your body disease free and best of all drinking these smoothies on a daily basis is keeping the doctor far far away!

These are the 18 secret superfoods and what they can do for your body and mind.

1. Avocado

Promotes the health of your heart

Avocado has wide ranging anti inflammatory benefits

Avocado supports cardiovascular health

Avocado promotes blood sugar regulation

Avocado has anti-cancer benefits

Avocados contains 18 amino acids that are required to form complete protein that is used more efficiently by your body than proteins that are found in meat foods

Avocados contain more natural fiber than any other fruit, and this high fiber content aids in digestion and total body absorption of nutrients

Healthy fats found in avocados do raise the "good" cholesterol while lowering the "bad" cholesterol and the triglycerides by 20%.

Avocados contain 35% more potassium than do bananas

Potassium is important because it regulates your blood pressure

Avocados do provide the lutein that is necessary to protect you from age related eye degeneration problems

The anti inflammatory properties of avocado fruits do prevent and do treat rheumatoid arthritis

Sufficient amounts of oleic acid also do improve your cardiovascular system and do protect you against prostate and breast cancer

Glutathione that is contained in avocados boosts your immune system and does keep your nervous system healthy and fit

Avocado health benefits are also considered one of the nature's most effective moisturizers for the skin

Avocado has shown to increase collagen production of the skin as well as reduce the size and appearance of wrinkles

Avocado Beauty Tips:

Mix the pulp of an avocado and apply it as a masque directly to your face and body skin

If you suffer from sunburn, eczema, dry spots or psoriasis, the healthy fat in avocado protects, repairs and moisturizes your skin

The pulp closest to the avocado skin has the highest concentration of nutrients

Make sure to use this pulp and scrape it off the skin

Apply this pulp directly to the skin for a soft and a supple result

2. Blueberries

These are the benefits of blueberries:

Whole body antioxidant support

Cardiovascular benefits

Cognitive benefits

Blood sugar benefits

Eye health

Anti cancer benefits

3. Coconut

These are the benefits of coconut:

Helps prevent obesity

Improves heart health

High in dietary fiber

Low glycemic index

www.facebook.com/healthysmoothiesrecipes

Reduces sweet cravings

Improves digestion

Quick energy boost

In addition, coconut contains no trans fats, is gluten free, non toxic, hypoallergenic

It also contains antiviral, antibacterial, antifungal, and anti parasitic healing properties

Coconut helps your overall immune system functions

4. Ginger

These are the benefits of ginger:

Gastrointestinal relief

Safe and effective relief of nausea

anti inflammatory effects

Protection against colorectal cancer

Ginger induces cell death in ovarian cancer cells

Immune boosting action

5. Kale

These are the benefits of kale:

Antioxidant related health benefits

Anti inflammatory health benefits

Glucosinolates and cancer preventive benefits

Glucosinolates in kale and their detox activating isothiocyanates

Cardiovascular support

Other health related benefits

6. Raspberries

These are the benefits of raspberries:

Antioxidant and anti inflammatory benefits

Obesity and blood sugar benefits

Anti cancer benefits

7. Papaya

These are the benefits of papaya:

Protection against heart disease

Anti inflammatory effects

Promotes digestive health

Immune support

Protection against rheumatoid arthritis

Papaya and green tea in combination prevents prostate cancer

8. Broccoli

These are the benefits of broccoli:

The cancer-inflammation-oxidative stress-detox connection

anti Inflammatory benefits

antioxidant benefits

broccoli can enhance detoxification

broccoli and cancer prevention

broccoli and digestive support

broccoli and cardiovascular support

9. Apricot

These are the benefits of apricot:

Apricots do protect your eyesight

Apricots do contain nutrients (vitamin A for good vision and it is also a powerful antioxidant, Vitamin A quenches the free radical damage to cells and tissues)

10. Banana

These are the benefits of bananas:

Cardiovascular protection from potassium and fiber

soothing protection from ulcers

improving elimination

protect your eyesight

build better bones with bananas

Bananas do promote kidney health through regular and moderate intake

11. Pecan Nuts

These are the benefits of pecan nuts:

One of the most significant facts of pecan nutrition is that pecans are the best antioxidants

Pecan nuts help preventing coronary heart diseases

Pecan nuts contain vitamin E which is a natural antioxidant that protects blood lipids from getting oxidized

Pecans have cholesterol lowering properties

The plant sterols in pecans have cholesterol lowering characteristics

Pecan nuts do help in weight loss

Pecans help in increasing the metabolic rate of the body and they do improve satiety

Pecans do contain 19 plus vitamins and minerals

Vitamins from the B group, vitamin A, vitamin E, calcium, potassium, folic acid, phosphorus, zinc, magnesium just to name a few

Pecans are rich source of proteins and contain less carbohydrates and zero cholesterol

Pecans are best suited for a sodium restricted diet and for heart patients as well as for people with high blood pressure because they are sodium free

www.facebook.com/healthysmoothiesrecipes

12. Walnuts

Walnuts have cardiovascular benefits

Walnuts help reduce problems in metabolic syndrome

Walnuts are beneficial in treatment of type 2 diabetes

Walnuts have anti cancer benefits

Walnuts have anti inflammatory nutrients which is perfect for the support of your bone health

A large amount of walnuts decreases your blood levels of N-telopeptides of type 1 collagen

Walnuts are a desirable food for support of weight loss and for prevention of obesity

Walnuts are unique in their collection of anti inflammatory nutrients

These nutrients include omega 3 fatty acids

Walnuts also promote anti cancer benefits

13. Carrots

Carrots have a rich supply of antioxidant nutrients called beta carotene

These delicious orange vegetables are the source not only of beta carotene, but also of a wide variety of antioxidants plus other health supporting nutrients.

Other benefits of carrots:

Antioxidant benefits

Cardiovascular benefits

Vision health

14. Lemon

Lemons are very alkalizing for the body and they do help to restore the balance of the pH

Lemons are rich in flavonoids and vitamin C

Vitamin C works against infections like colds and the flu

Lemons are a wonderful stimulation to your liver

Lemon is a dissolvent of uric acid and other poisons

It is a is a great liver detoxifier

It cleanses your bowels

Lemons increase peristalsis in the bowels

The citric acid in lemon juice helps to dissolve calcium deposits, gallstones and kidney stones

Vitamin C in lemons helps the body to neutralize free radicals that are linked to most types of diseases and aging

Lemon peel contains phytonutrient tangeretin

Phytonutrient Tangeretin has been proven to be effective for brain disorders (Parkinson disease for example)

Lemons destroy intestinal worms

In a condition of insufficient oxygen and breathing problems (mountain climbing, etc.) lemons are very helpful

Some other helpful facts about lemons:

Scurvy is treated by giving 1-2 ounces of lemon juice with water every 2 to 4 hours

Tip:

Mix the juice of one lemon or lime to warm water and drink this mixture first thing in the morning to start your day

15. Peanuts

These are the benefits of peanuts:

Peanuts are a rich source of antioxidants

Heart health benefits

Potentially reduced risk of strokes

Helps prevent gallstones

Protects against Alzheimer and other age related cognitive decline health problems

Lowers risk of weight gain

16. Cinnamon

Anti-clotting actions

Anti-microbial activity

Blood sugar control

Cinnamon's scent boosts the brain function

Calcium and fiber improve colon health and protect against heart disease

Cinnamon is a traditional warming remedy

17. Pineapple

Potential Anti inflammatory and digestive benefits

Antioxidant protection and immune support

Protection against macular degeneration

My Favorite Smoothie Quote

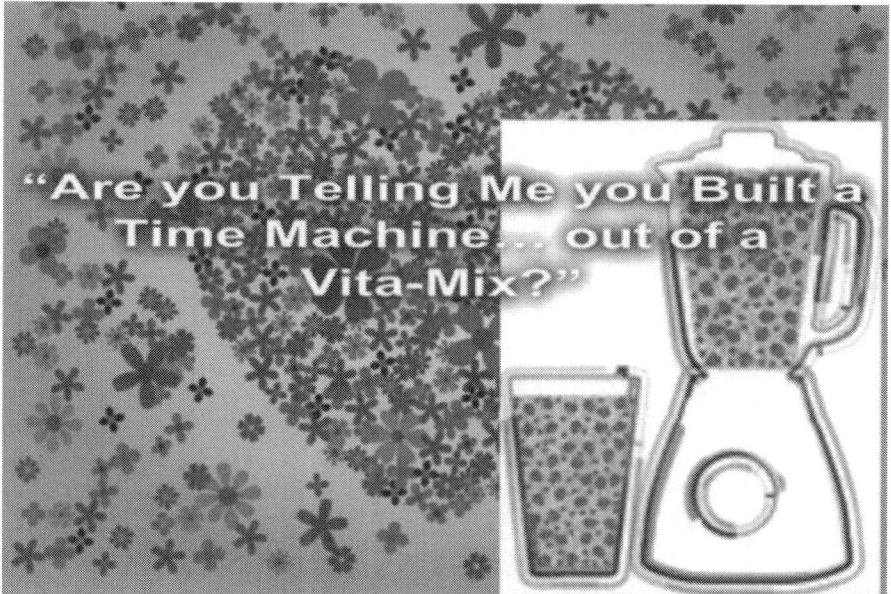

www.facebook.com/healthysmoothierecipes

My Personal Rules For Weight Loss With These Smoothies

Blend a couple of times a day and as long as you plan to apply your Smoothie diet.

Combine it with eating healthy clean foods for 1 meal and a healthy snack or two throughout the day.

Combine your smoothie diet with a light daily workout ritual like Yoga or any other physical activity.

The more smoothies you drink during the day and the less processed foods you consume the more weight you are going to lose.

Don't push yourself too hard. This is a long term strategy and once you reached your dieting goal, make sure to include these healthy smoothies into your daily meal plan in order to stay fit and keep a lean body.

Smoothie 1: Strawberry N'Creams

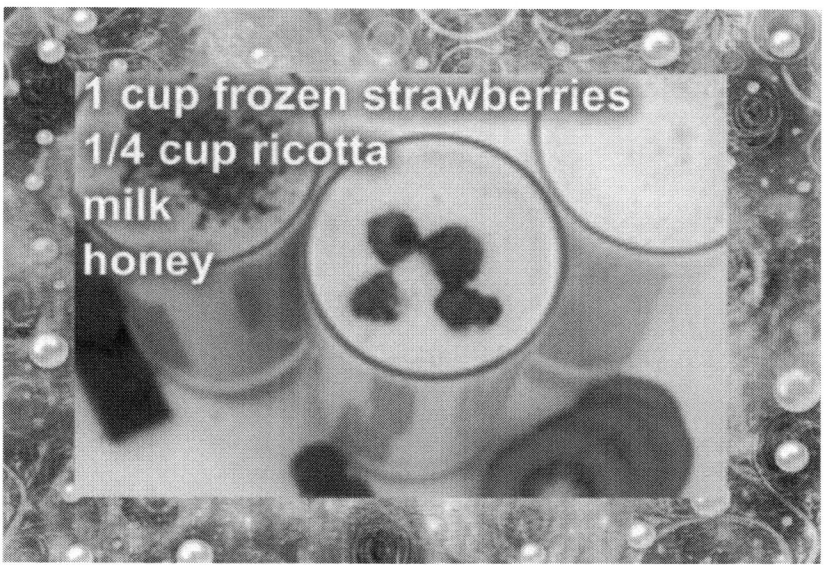

"Show Me The Smoothies!" Famous Smoothie Quote

If you love tasty smoothies with some strange secret ingredients that are heavenly deliciously then you might consider the Strawberry n'Creams smoothie.

Imagine the best of creams and cheeses combined with some zesty red fruits like strawberries or raspberries.

Pouring the contents of a delightful fruit-cream-cheese platter into your favorite blender (in my case I am using the Vitamix) and whip it all together into a creamy delight.

www.facebook.com/healthysmoothierecipes

This cheese, cream and strawberry smoothie drink contains the following ingredients:

Ingredients:

1 cup frozen raspberries or strawberries whatever you prefer or have available

1/4 cup of fresh organic Italian ricotta cheese

1/2 cup of milk or skim milk (depending on your goals and if you are on a diet just use the skim milk and do not add the rich cream)

A Dash of rich tasty cream to swirl this into a creamy and rich tasting delight

Raw organic Honey (optional and to your taste)

Directions:

For all these Smoothie recipe simply follow my 5 minute directions. Add all the ingredients into your Vitamix or similar high-speed blender. Make sure to add fresh spring water. Add as much water as you like in order to reach your desired thickness of the smoothie. For all the smoothie recipes, make sure to use organic products, fruits and vegetables if possible.

Mix the strawberries, the ricotta cheese, the milk and the cream in a blender and swirl it into a creamy texture while adding the raw honey.

In the summer adding some additional ice cubes might be a very very refreshing idea. Instead of the ice cubes you can also add some strawberry or raspberry sherbert or ice cream.

www.facebook.com/healthysmoothiesrecipes

This is totally optional and depends on your goal. If your goal is to lose weight then just skip the creamy stuff!

Enjoy this refreshing and delicious smoothie!

Smoothie 2: Mango/Papaya Protein Booster

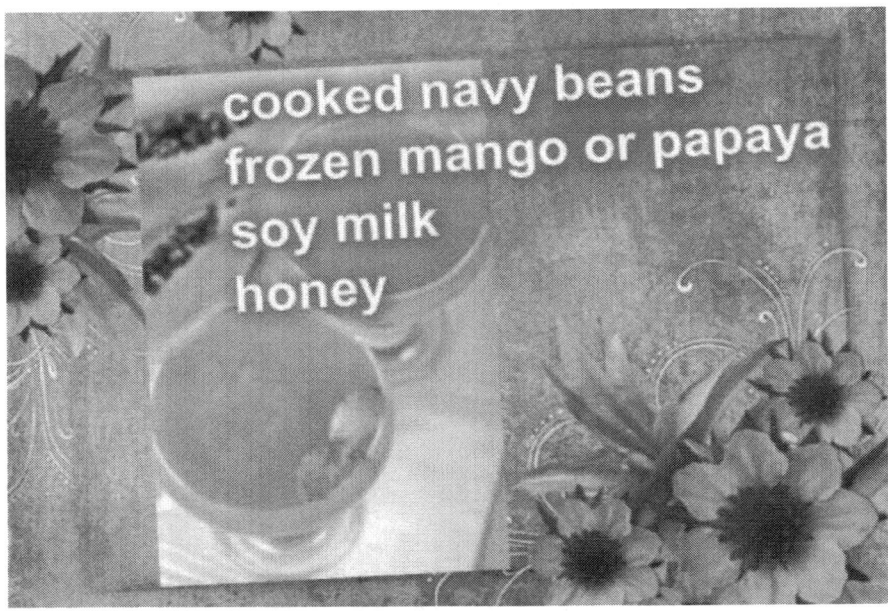

"Next Time, Indiana Jones, it will Take More Than Smoothies to Save You." Famous Smoothie Quote

A combination of healthy and lean making protein and mango is what this smoothie is all about. The Mango Protein booster is perfect if your goal is to follow a lean and clean smoothie diet.

So what is the secret of this protein booster?

Usually smoothies are well known for their high protein content because they do rely on protein powder.

The secret ingredient fot the Mango Protein booster however is the protein of the cooked navy beans.

www.facebook.com/healthysmoothiesrecipes

You might not like the idea of combining beans into your smoothies, but I am going to change your paradigm quickly after you had your first serving.

I have tested this smoothie with a lot of smoothie lovers before adding it to my collection. I am constantly testing and proving new smoothie recipes that I am gradually adding to my "Tested & Proven Smoothie Recipe Collection"

This one has passed the test because it is not only delicious, but it is such a health treat and perfect for you if you are trying to lose weight with smoothies.

Between the navy beans and the soy milk that is included in this smoothie, you are going to consume around ten to eleven grams of pure protein.

This protein rich smoothie drink contains the following ingredients:

Ingredients:

1/3 cup of cooked navy beans (organic if possible)

1-1/2 cups of frozen papaya or mango

3/4 cups of organic soy milk

2 teaspoons of raw honey (this is optional and try organic raw honey if you can)

Directions:

For all these Smoothie recipe simply follow my 5 minute directions. Add all the ingredients into your Vitamix or similar high-speed blender. Make sure to add fresh spring water if needed. Add as much water as you like in order to reach your desired thickness of the smoothie.

For all the smoothie recipes, make sure to use organic products, fruits and vegetables if possible.

Mix the cooked navy beans and the tropical frozen fruits (mango or papaya) together and process them in your high speed blender until both ingredients are well combined together. Next, add the organic soy milk and the raw honey and continue mixing until everything is combined into a nice and creamy texture. Add ice if needed and to your own liking.

You can adjust the raw organic honey to your preference or you can skip this step if you do not have a sweet tooth or if you are following a strict smoothie diet with unsweetened smoothies.

www.facebook.com/healthysmoothiesrecipes

Smoothie 3: Superfood Greens Shake

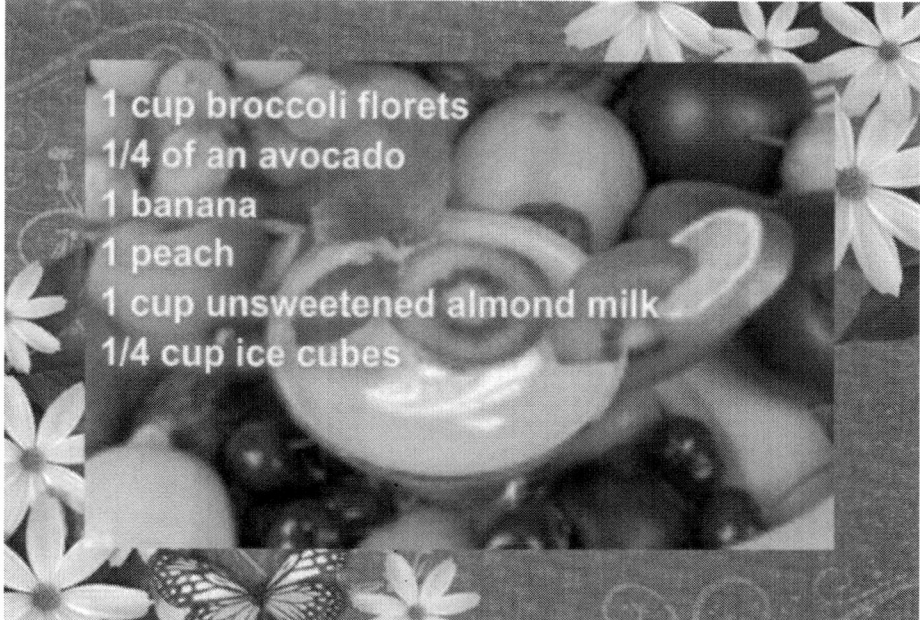

"Round up the Usual Fruits and Vegetables."

A fortified and nutritious combination of healthy and lean making superfood greens like broccoli and avocado.

This lean Superfood Greens Shake gets its rich flavour from the nutty tasting avocado.

Who says that vegetables are for lunch and dinner only? This lean green cocktail contains delicious and zesty fruits that are swirled into the greens and this smoothie makes for a perfect wholesome and healthy start of your day so that you do not need to wait for lunchtime to eat these healthy veggies.

www.facebook.com/healthysmoothierecipes

This Superfood Greens Shake contains the following ingredients:

Ingredients:

1/4 of an organic avocado

1 cup of organic broccoli florets

1 peeled and organic banana that is already chopped and frozen

1 organic chopped peach or apricot or nectarine

1 cup of unsweetened and organic almond milk

ice cubes to your liking

Directions:

For all these Smoothie recipe simply follow my 5 minute directions. Add all the ingredients into your Vitamix or similar high-speed blender. Make sure to add fresh spring water or ice cubes if needed. Add as much water as you like in order to reach your desired thickness of the smoothie. For all the smoothie recipes, make sure to use organic products, fruits and vegetables if possible.

Mix all the ingredients together and process them with your favorite blender until all of the ingredients are well combined together. Make sure the broccoli is broken down and all the other ingredients are well swirled together in a rich looking creamy texture.

You can add more organic almond milk, water, or ice cubes (depending on your goal) if you like a more fluid and water downed smoothie. If you like you can also add some raw honey or if you are on a smoothie diet and like it sweet you can add a little bit of your favourite sweetener.

Other people love the unsweetened taste!

www.facebook.com/healthysmoothierecipes

Smoothie 4: Exotic Coconut & Green Superpower Ginger Smoothie

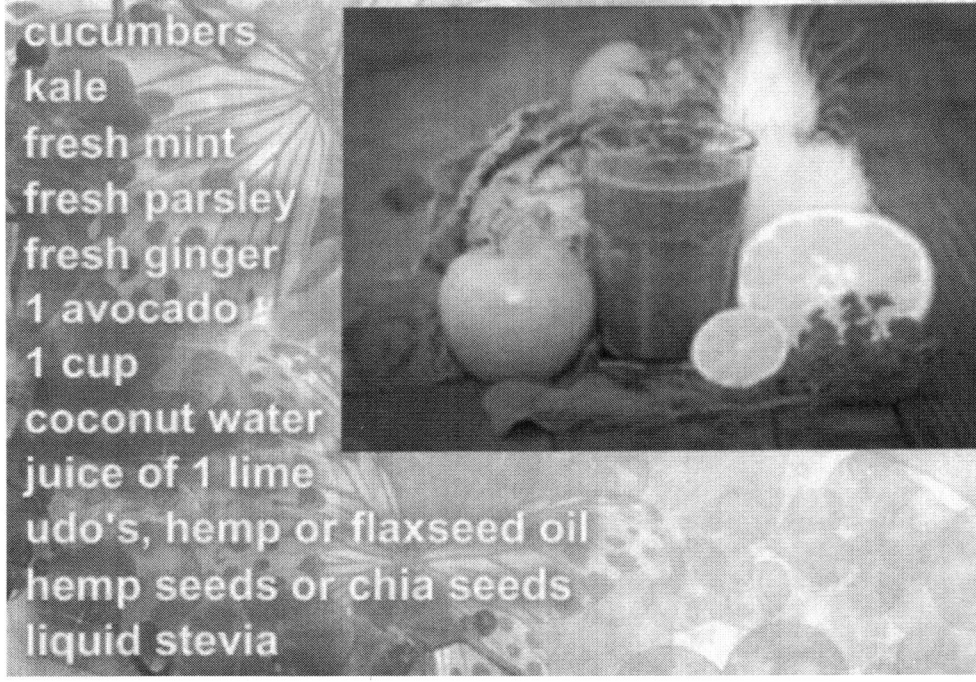

cucumbers
kale
fresh mint
fresh parsley
fresh ginger
1 avocado
1 cup coconut water
juice of 1 lime
udo's, hemp or flaxseed oil
hemp seeds or chia seeds
liquid stevia

"Not that I loved Caesar Salads Less, but that I loved Green Smoothies More"

Let's talk about a powerful combination of some fortified, exotic and nutritious superfoods like cucumbers, kale, mint, ginger, coconut water, parsley and more.

The secret ingredient that I use here in order to bring out a rich nutty and exotic tasting flavour is the coconut water.

www.facebook.com/healthysmoothiesrecipes

This is a magical mixture of green and exotic superfoods that are healing in nature. These are ingredients that do not only taste deliciously and exotically, but they will give your body and brain the most nutritious and beneficial nourishment.

Coconut is especially beneficial to help prevent obesity and it improves the heart health.

Coconut is high in dietary fiber, it has a low glycemic index, it reduces sweet cravings, it improves digestion.

It is also a quick energy booster.

In addition, coconut contains no trans fats, it is gluten free and it is non toxic and hypoallergenic.

It also contains antiviral, antibacterial, antifungal, and anti parasitic healing properties.

Coconut helps your overall immune system functions.

Ginger is helping with gastrointestinal relief.

Safe and effective relief of nausea and vomiting during pregnancy.

Ginger carries anti inflammatory effects and helps protect against colorectal cancer.

Ginger induces cell death in ovarian cancer cells and helps boost the immune system.

The Exotic & Green Superpower Smoothie with coconut and ginger contains the following ingredients:

Ingredients:

1-2 organic small cucumbers

3 medium kale leaves (torn)

5 stems of fresh mint

3 stems of fresh parsley

2.5 cm pieces of fresh organic ginger

1 organic avocado

1 cup of organic coconut water

juice of 1 lime

1-2 teaspoons of udo's, hemp or flaxseed oil (optional)

1-2 tablespoons of hemp seeds or chia seeds (optional)

2 - 3 drops of liquid stevia

Directions:

For all these Smoothie recipe simply follow my 5 minute directions. Add all the ingredients into your Vitamix or similar high-speed blender. Make sure to add fresh spring water or ice cubes if needed. Add as much water as you like in order to reach your desired thickness of the smoothie. For all the smoothie recipes, make sure to use organic products, fruits and vegetables if possible.

Mix all the ingredients together and process them with your favorite blender until all of the ingredients are well combined together. Make sure the broccoli is broken down and all the other ingredients are well swirled together in a rich looking creamy texture.

Add a little filtered spring water or ice cubes if needed for your desired consistency.

www.facebook.com/healthysmoothiesrecipes

If you like you can also add some raw honey or if you are on a smoothie diet and like it sweet you can add a little bit of your favorite sweetener.

Other people love the unsweetened taste!

www.facebook.com/healthysmoothierecipes

Smoothie 5: Rich Berry Screamer

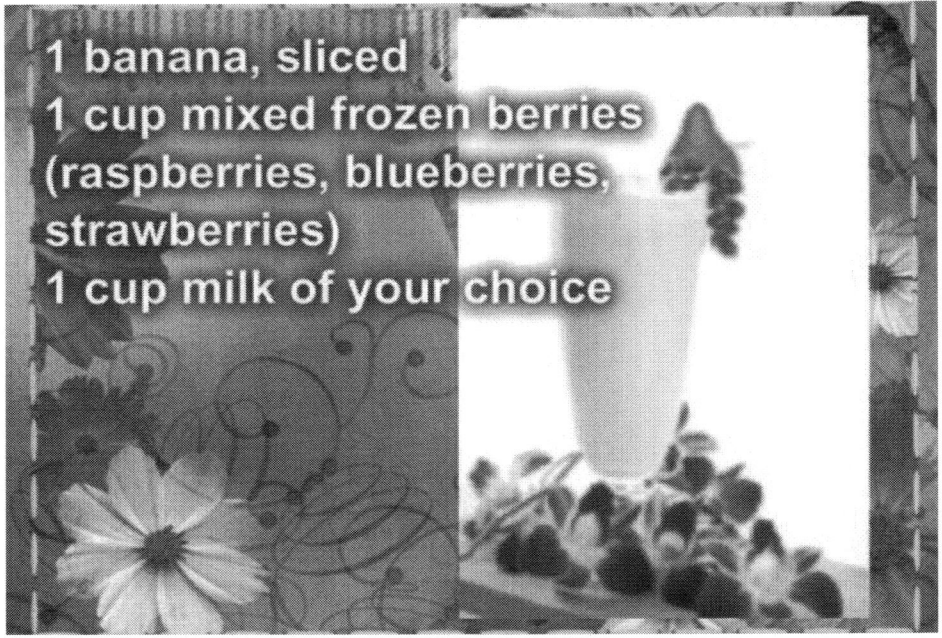

"Are you Telling Me you Built a Time Machine… out of a Vita-Mix?"

This is a refreshing blend of red, blue and black berries with or without a tropical twist.

It is a great hydratation solution and thirst quencher after a physical workout.

The Rich Berry Screamer Smoothie contains the following ingredients:

Ingredients:

1 small organic banana (sliced)

1 cup of mixed frozen berries (raspberries, blueberries, blackberries, strawberries)

1 cup milk of your choice (skim if you are on a smoothie diet)

Tropical orange twist:

Nothing welcomes warmer weather better than the twist of a tropical inspired flavor from pineapples and citrus fruits like oranges and limes.

fresh orange juice

twist of lime or lemon

fresh pinapple juice

Directions:

For all these Smoothie recipe simply follow my 5 minute directions. Add all the ingredients into your Vitamix or similar high-speed blender. Make sure to add fresh spring water or ice cubes if needed. Add as much water as you like in order to reach your desired thickness of the smoothie. For all the smoothie recipes, make sure to use organic products, fruits and vegetables if possible.

Mix all the ingredients together and process them with your favorite blender until all of the ingredients are well combined together. Add a little filtered spring water or ice cubes if needed for your desired consistency.

Add all the ingredients to your blender and puree the mixture until everything is smooth.

www.facebook.com/healthysmoothierecipes

www.facebook.com/healthysmoothiesrecipes

Smoothie 6: Vanilla Smoothie Delight

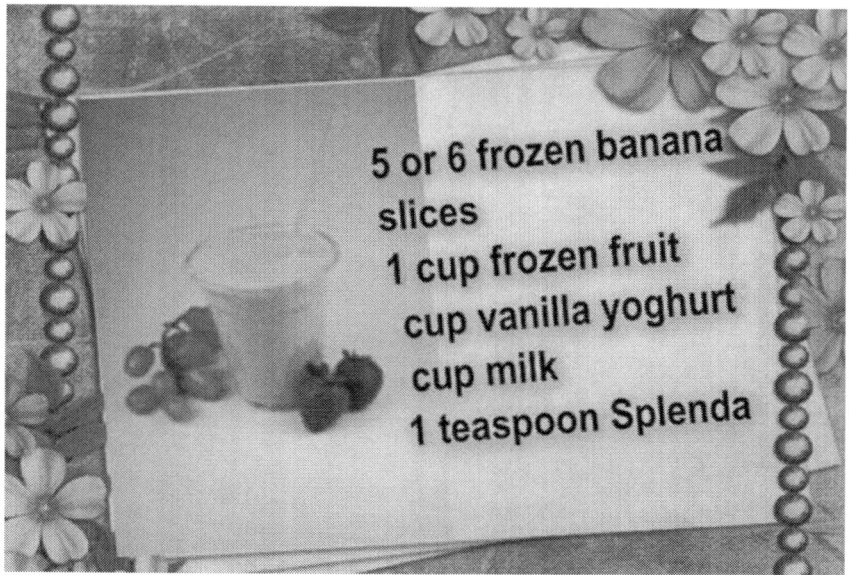

"A Green Smoothie is Worth a Thousand Donuts"

A smoothie might be in the blended beverage category, but a smoothie certainly represent very different aspects.

I love the creamy and delicious taste of a smoothie combined with the health benefits that are offered by a smoothie.

All you need is one very secret ingredient that provides the body and brain with a very powerful health benefit and you can turn a simple milkshake into a nutritious drink.

www.facebook.com/healthysmoothierecipes

In the case of the Vanilla Smoothie Delight the secret ingredient are frozen bananas.

Did you know that when bananas are frozen and then blended down, they take on the texture of real ice cream?

Yes, real ice cream but without all the dangerous and sick making additives and fats.

In this case I suggest to buy a whole whack of fresh organic bananas. Let them sit out until they have ripened nicely and are yellow.

They should also show some brown spots, but not have gone quite so far as to be in banana bread making material.

Peel your bananas and slice them so that each slice is about 1.5 to 2 centimeters thick.

Separate all the banana slices and lay them flat in a Ziploc bag and place them like this in your freezer.

Avoid throwing them all in at once. They may be hard to break apart in the quantities that you need them later when they are in a frozen condition. Once you have gone through this freezing process, you will have bananas on hand for your smoothie delights for a good amount of time.

This will be a huge time saver because you can live healthy without having to go to the store and buy fresh bananas all the time.

The Vanilla Smoothie Delight is a great smoothie for beginners and you can play around with it and add some of your own variations.

www.facebook.com/healthysmoothiesrecipes

Make sure to write down your own ingredients that you like to add and your preparation method so that you will remember it later.

I suggest using a site like Evernote or a mobile app where you can quickly take all your notes for later reference.

The Vanilla Smoothie Delight is a great recipe that can act as a base for you to build from and it contains the following ingredients:

Ingredients:

5 or 6 small frozen banana slices (organic if possible)

1 cup of frozen fruits (be creative with your selection like peaches, apricots, strawberries, blueberries, blackberries, raspberries, papaya, mango. Make sure the fruits are frozen because this will add to the creamy texture of the smoothie)

¼ cup of organic vanilla yoghurt

½ cup of milk (skim if you are on a strict smoothie diet)

raw honey or splenda (optional and to your liking)

Directions:

For all these Smoothie recipe simply follow my 5 minute directions. Add all the ingredients into your Vitamix or similar high-speed blender. Make sure to add fresh spring water or ice cubes if needed. Add as much water as you like in order to reach your desired thickness of the smoothie. For all the smoothie recipes, make sure to use organic products, fruits and vegetables if possible.

www.facebook.com/healthysmoothierecipes

Mix all the ingredients together and process them with your favorite blender until all of the ingredients are well combined together. Blend the frozen slices of bananas and fruits in your favorite blender or food processor on high speed.

You may need to stop occasionally with the process and return some of the fruits to the base of the blender as the fruits can quickly creep up the sides of your mixing bowl.

Keep blending until all the fruits are broken down into a nice smoothie texture.

Next, add in the vanilla yoghurt, the milk and the raw honey or splenda and continue to mix the drink until thoroughly swirled together.

Transfer your drink to a large glass or two smaller ones and enjoy your delicious and nutritious Vanilla Smoothie Delight.

If you need you can also add some more ice cubes or a little filtered spring water depending on your desired consistency.

www.facebook.com/healthysmoothiesrecipes

Smoothie 7: Purple Power Booster

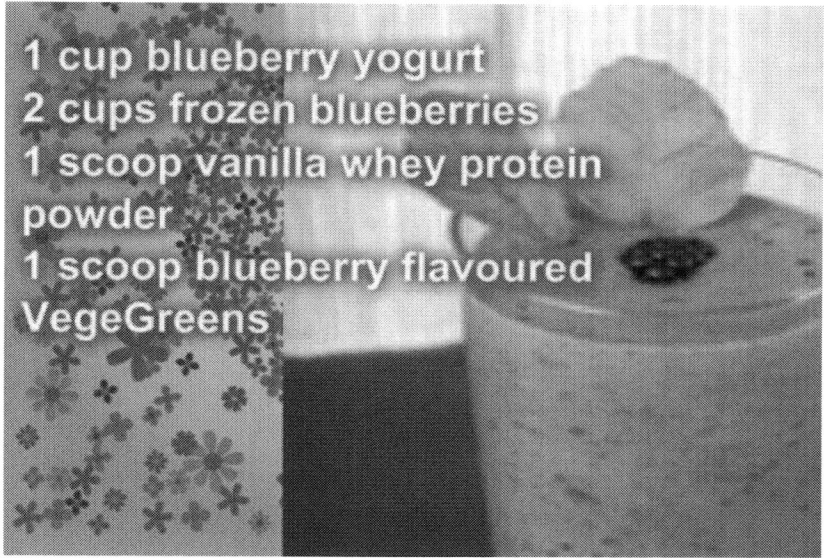

"All Right, Mr. DeMille, I'm Ready for my Purple Smoothie."

Start your day with a smooth start and loading up on lots of protein is a beneficial way to start your day. This smoothie will also give your muscles the perfect energy they need after a tough workout. This smoothie will provide your body with all the nutrients and fuel that it requires.

This protein packed smoothie is loaded with minerals and vitamins. The amount of protein will give you every ounce of energy that you need each and every day.

The Purple Power Booster contains the following ingredients:

Ingredients:

1 cup of purple/blue or vanilla yogurt (blueberry if possible but you can also use vanilla yogurt)

2 cups of frozen purple fruits like blueberries because they are turning this smoothie into a superfood smoothie

1 scoop of vanilla whey protein powder

1 scoop of blueberry flavoured VegeGreens

2 cups of fresh spring water

Directions:

For all these Smoothie recipe simply follow my 5 minute directions. Add all the ingredients into your Vitamix or similar high-speed blender. Make sure to add fresh spring water or ice cubes if needed. Add as much water as you like in order to reach your desired thickness of the smoothie. For all the smoothie recipes, make sure to use organic products, fruits and vegetables if possible.

Mix all the ingredients together and process them with your favorite blender until all of the ingredients are well combined together. Mix all ingredients thoroughly in a food processor or blender.

Add a little filtered spring water or ice cubes if needed for your desired consistency.

Transfer the delicious mix in your favorite smoothie glasses and enjoy.

www.facebook.com/healthysmoothiesrecipes

If you like you can also add some raw honey or if you are on a smoothie diet and like it sweet you can add a little bit of your favorite sweetener.

Some people love the unsweetened and more natural taste.

www.facebook.com/healthysmoothierecipes

Smoothie 8: Kefir Peanut Butter Breakfast Smoothie

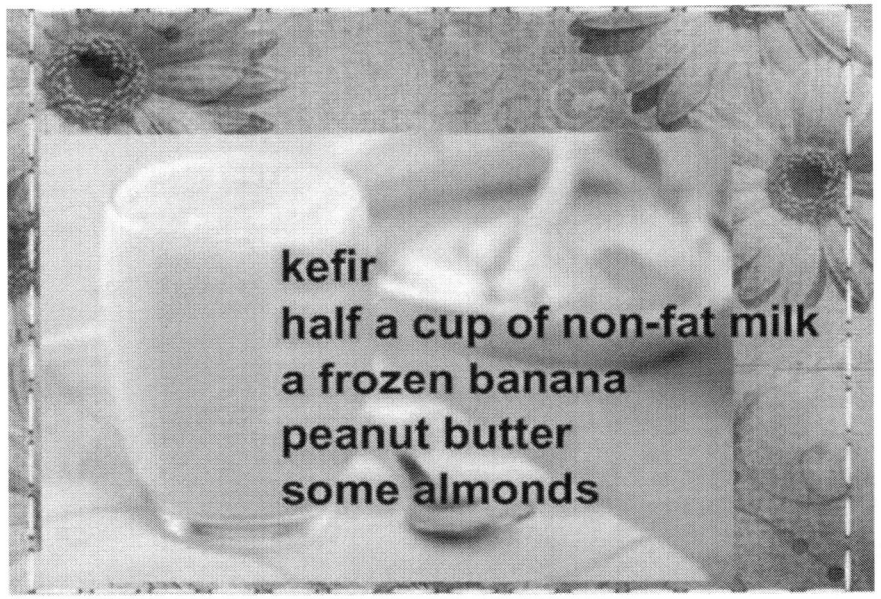

kefir
half a cup of non-fat milk
a frozen banana
peanut butter
some almonds

"What's in a Name? That which we call a Green Smoothie By any Other Name would Taste as Sweet."

This smoothie contains some beneficial ingredients like almonds and kefir.

Almonds are some powerful miracle workers. They are high in potassium. They also boost your brain activity, reduce the risk of a heart attack and the lower bad cholesterol.

Breakfast is the most important meal of the day.

Make sure not to skip it and consume this powerful breakfast smoothie instead.

This breakfast smoothie is a great way to incorporate nutrition into your day and start your day in an energized and stress free way.

This smoothie delivers a drink that is full of fiber, good carbs and healthy nutrients.

If your goal is to lose weight, I highly recommend to consume this highly nutritionally dense breakfast smoothie every morning during your smoothie diet. It will help you lose weight, keep lean, stave off illnesses, keep clean and boost energy.

This Kefir Peanut Butter Breakfast Smoothie contains the following ingredients:

Ingredients:

1 cup of kefir

some peanut butter for a nutty rich taste

1 organic small banana

a quarter cup of fresh pineapple

1 cup of organic almond milk (self made or bought)

www.facebook.com/healthysmoothierecipes

Directions:

For all these Smoothie recipe simply follow my 5 minute directions. Add all the ingredients into your Vitamix or similar high-speed blender. Make sure to add fresh spring water if needed. Add as much water as you like in order to reach your desired thickness of the smoothie. For all the smoothie recipes, make sure to use organic products, fruits and vegetables if possible.

Blend a cup of organic kefir, the peanut butter, a ripe banana, a quarter cup of fresh pineapple and one cup of almond milk and swirl it into a smooth silky treat.

Add ice if needed and to your own liking.

You can adjust some raw organic honey to your preference (if it is not sweat enough for your taste) or you can skip this step if you do not have a sweet tooth.

If you are following a strict smoothie diet, I recommend to keep the Smoothie unsweetened.

If the pineapple is ripe, it will add sugar in a natural way.

Smoothie 9: Blueberry Pecan & Vanilla Smoothie

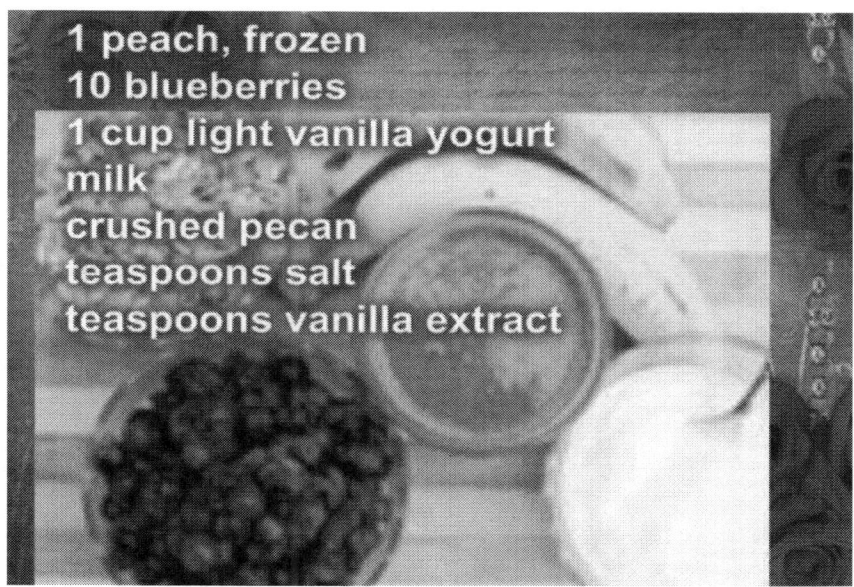

"Round up the Usual Fruits and Vegetables."

The Blueberry Pecan & Vanilla Smoothie is a combination of healthy and lean making superfood ingredients.

So what is the secret of this protein booster?

The secret ingredients are the pecans.

Pecan nuts are a very rich source of energy. Pecans do provide 690 calories / 100 g and do contain health benefiting nutrients: antioxidants, minerals, and vitamins. These are all essential for our wellness.

A regular intake of pecan nuts into your diet plan helps you to decrease total as well as LDL or otherwise known as "bad cholesterol". Eating these nuts does help the increase of HDL or otherwise known as the "good cholesterol" levels in your blood.

Studies also have shown that these healthy compounds that are contained in pecan nuts do in fact help the body remove toxic oxygen free radicals.

This helps protect the body from damages and diseases, infections and cancers.

Pecan nuts do contain anti proliferative properties of ellagic acid which is helping protect the human body from cancers.

Pecan nuts are also an excellent source of vitamin E. Especially rich in gamma tocopherol.

Vitamin E is a powerful lipid soluble antioxidant which is required for maintaining the integrity of cell membrane and Vitamin E helps protect the skin from harmful oxygen free radicals.

These tasty nuts are also a very rich sources of several important B-complex groups of vitamins which are needed for the enzyme metabolism inside the body.

Pecans also do provide a very rich source of minerals like potassium, manganese, calcium, magnesium, iron, magnesium, selenium and zinc.

I recommend to add a hand full of pecans into your smoothies every day to provide your body with sufficient levels of protein, minerals and vitamins.

This protein rich Blueberry Pecan & Vanilla Smoothie contains the following ingredients:

Ingredients:

1 organic peach (frozen)

10-20 organic blueberries (frozen)

1 cup light and fat free organic vanilla yogurt (frozen)

1/2 cup of milk or skim milk

1/2 tablespoon of crushed pecans

1/2 teaspoon of salt

1/4 teaspoons of organic vanilla extract

Directions:

For all these Smoothie recipe simply follow my 5 minute directions. Add all the ingredients into your Vitamix or similar high-speed blender. Make sure to add fresh spring water if needed. Add as much water as you like in order to reach your desired thickness of the smoothie. For all the smoothie recipes, make sure to use organic products, fruits and vegetables if possible.

Put all ingredients into your favorite blender. Blend the mix until your preferred smoothie consistency is reached!

Add ice if needed and to your own liking. You can also add some raw organic honey to your liking or you can skip this step if you do not have a sweet tooth. If you are following a strict smoothie diet, keep the smoothie in its natural and unsweetened form.

www.facebook.com/healthysmoothiesrecipes

Smoothie 10: Avocado Banana Berry Avalanche

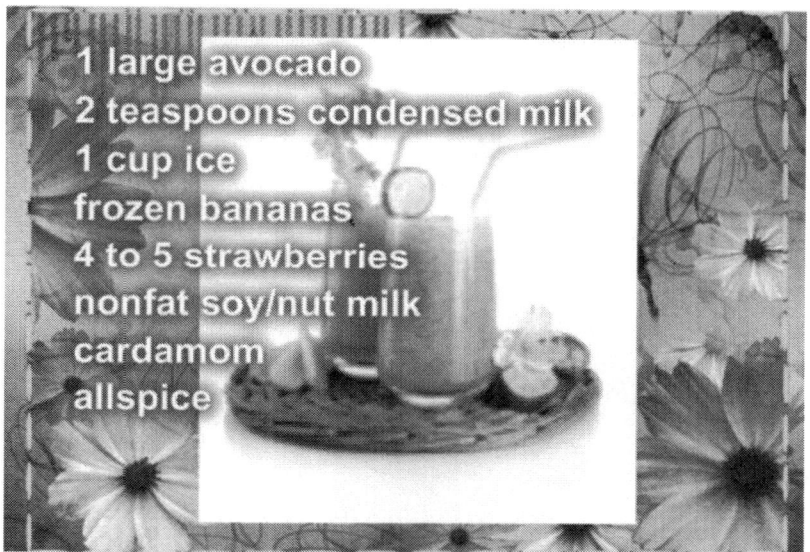

1 large avocado
2 teaspoons condensed milk
1 cup ice
frozen bananas
4 to 5 strawberries
nonfat soy/nut milk
cardamom
allspice

"You had me at 'Green Smoothie." Famous Smoothie Quote

A combination of healthy and lean making avocado and strawberries is what this smoothie's secret is all about.

The avocado is a superfood and strawberries are nutrient-rich and packed with antioxidants. Strawberries provide the body with a rich source of vitamin C and a wide range of health benefits.

Strawberries for example help with wrinkle prevention.

The Mayan Indians have a saying: "Where avocados grow, hunger or malnutrition has no friends."

www.facebook.com/healthysmoothierecipes

This antioxidant-rich avocado fruit enhances your heart's health, lowers your cholesterol and improves your skin.

Avocados are abundant in minerals and in vitamins.

Avocados contain beta-carotene, vitamins B6, lutein, vitamins C, E and K, zinc, selenium, potassium, folate, glutathione and omega 3 fatty acids.

These are just a few nutrients that are found in a single avocado.

This Avocado Banana Berry Avalanche is the perfect energy booster if your goal is to follow a lean and clean smoothie diet.

This Avocado Banana Berry Avalanche contains the following ingredients:

Avocado Beauty Recipe:

Mash the pulp of the avocado and apply it directly as a masque to your skin. Avocado contains some of the best anti aging antioxidants and amino acids used in many expensive brand beauty products.

If you suffer from dry skin, spots, sunburn, eczema, or psoriasis, the healthy fat that is contained in avocados is very beneficial for your skin and beauty care because it will heal you from distress, inflammation, dry skin and it will also protect your skin from more damages in the future.

The oil that comes from avocados is the closest to the natural skin oil that is produced by the human body and you can use the avocado pulp and put it on your skin because it has the highest concentration of nutrients.

Just apply it directly to the skin for a soft and supple result.

Ingredients:

1 large organic avocado

2 teaspoons of condensed milk

1 to 1 1/2 frozen organic bananas

5 to 8 frozen or fresh strawberries

a splash of organic non fat soy or other organic nut milk

a pinch of cardamom

a pinch of allspice

ice cubes

Directions:

For all these Smoothie recipe simply follow my 5 minute directions. Add all the ingredients into your Vitamix or similar high-speed blender. Make sure to add fresh spring water if needed. Add as much water as you like in order to reach your desired thickness of the smoothie. For all the smoothie recipes, make sure to use organic products, fruits and vegetables if possible.

Scoop out the avocado fruit into your favorite high speed blender. Add 2 teaspoons of condensed milk. Add the ice cubes and blend all together until you get a a semi creamy and silky texture.

Next add the bananas, the strawberries and the organic non fat soy or nut milk. Finally add the cardamom and the allspice and blend until you reach your desired texture.

www.facebook.com/healthysmoothierecipes

I prefer mine very smooth, but some people who tested it preferred a chewable texture of this smoothie. You can always add some more ice cubes or fresh spring water to your liking to get the perfect texture.

Smoothie 11: Hazel Banana Vanilla Walnut Cream Smoothie

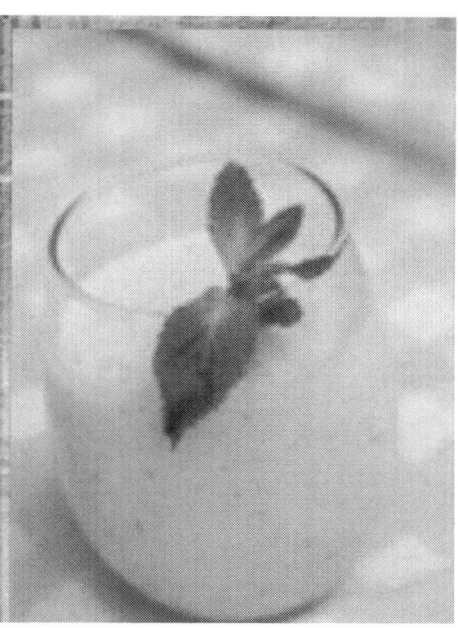

4 medium bananas
light brown sugar
hazelnuts
1/4 cups milk
1/4 cups dark rum
or hazelnut liqueur
banana liqueur
vanilla syrup
half and half
ice cubes
chopped walnuts

"Hazel Smoothies, I think this is the Beginning of a Beautiful Relationship."

Let's talk about a scrumptious smoothie called the Hazel Banana Vanilla Walnut Cream Smoothie.

It contains some tasty and nutty ingredients like hazelnuts, hazelnut liqueur, banana liqueur, vanilla syrup, and more tasty flavors.

I do not recommend this if you are on a strict smoothie diet, but if you want to treat yourself with a heavenly tasty delight, you must give this one a try.

www.facebook.com/healthysmoothierecipes

It contains the following ingredients:

Ingredients:

4 medium bananas (organic if possible and peeled, sliced into 1/2 inch slices)

6 tablespoons of light brown sugar (organic if possible)

1/4 cups of organic hazelnuts

1/4 cup of milk or skim milk

1/4 cups of dark rum or hazelnut liqueur (I prefer the hazelnut liqueur for the nutty taste!)

2 tablespoons of chopped hazelnuts (for the garnish and totally optional)

1 ounce of banana liqueur

1 ounce of vanilla syrup (organic if possible)

2 ounces of half and half

ice cubes

chopped organic walnuts

2 ounces of whipped cream (organic cream if possible)

Directions:

For all these Smoothie recipe simply follow my 5 minute directions. Add all the ingredients into your Vitamix or similar high-speed blender. Make sure to add fresh spring water or ice cubes if needed.

www.facebook.com/healthysmoothiesrecipes

Add as much water as you like in order to reach your desired thickness of the smoothie. For all the smoothie recipes, make sure to use organic products, fruits and vegetables if possible.

Place the sliced bananas in a sealed plastic bag and put them back in your freezer and let it freezer for one hour. Place the brown sugar and the hazelnuts in a blender and grind everything together until it is smooth.

Place the frozen bananas, the ice cubes, the milk, the rum or the hazelnut liqueur, the banana liqueur, the vanilla syrup and the half and half in the blender with the brown sugar.

Add ice and blend until smooth

Pour the smoothie drink into your favorite smoothie glasses. Garnish with a topping of whipped cream and sprinkle with chopped hazelnuts and walnuts and serve this tasty delight immediately.

Smoothie 12: The Beta Carotene Energy Booster

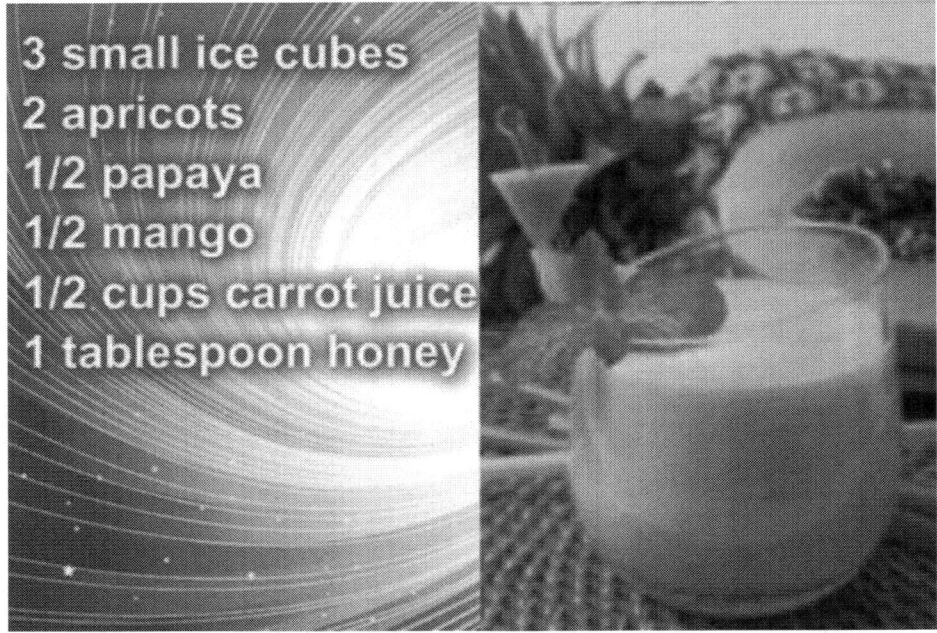

3 small ice cubes
2 apricots
1/2 papaya
1/2 mango
1/2 cups carrot juice
1 tablespoon honey

"May the Smoothie be with you...Always"

Let's talk about a powerful combination of some fortified, exotic and nutritious orange superfoods like carrots, papaya, mango and more.

The secret ingredient that I use here in order to bring out a rich nutty flavour of this smoothie is the carrot juice that contains a rich source of beta carotene.

This is a magical mixture of orange colored nutritious and healing vegetables and fruits. These are ingredients that do not only taste deliciously, but they will also give your body and brain the most powerful health benefits.

www.facebook.com/healthysmoothiesrecipes

Carrots have a rich supply of antioxidant nutrients called beta carotene.

These delicious orange vegetables are the source not only of beta carotene, but also of a wide variety of antioxidants plus other health supporting nutrients.

Other benefits of carrots are antioxidant benefits, cardiovascular benefits and vision for your health.

The Beta Carotene Energy Booster Smoothie contains the following ingredients:

Ingredients:

2 apricots (sliced and pitted)

1/2 papaya (frozen in chunks)

1/2 mango (frozen in chunks)

1/2 cups carrot juice

1 tablespoon of raw organic honey

3 small ice cubes

Option:

Fresh orange juice

Directions:

For all these Smoothie recipe simply follow my 5 minute directions. Add all the ingredients into your Vitamix or similar high-speed blender. Make sure to add fresh spring water or ice cubes if needed. Add as much water as you like in order to reach your desired thickness of the smoothie. For all the smoothie recipes, make sure to use organic products, fruits and vegetables if possible.

Mix all the ingredients in the order listed together and process them with your favorite high speed blender until all of the ingredients are well combined together. Make sure that everything is broken down and all the ingredients are well swirled together in a rich looking orangy colored texture.

Add the raw honey and blend a few more seconds.

Serve the smoothie in a frosted glass.

Option: If you like a thinner consistency, you can add some fresh orange juice. Add the orange juice and blend everything for one more time.

www.facebook.com/healthysmoothiesrecipes

Smoothie 13: The Blackberry Blueberry Blue Preserve Energy Triangle

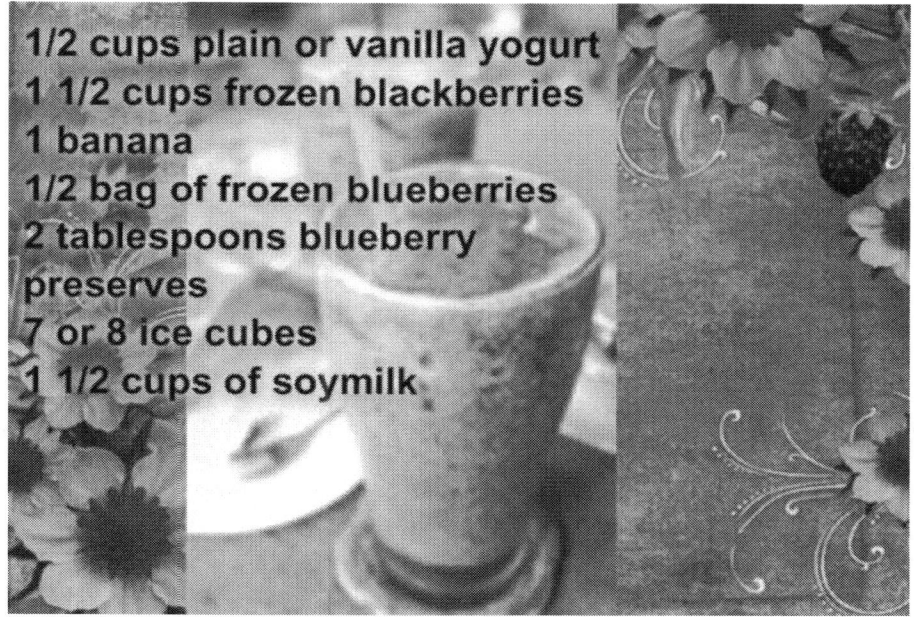

1/2 cups plain or vanilla yogurt
1 1/2 cups frozen blackberries
1 banana
1/2 bag of frozen blueberries
2 tablespoons blueberry preserves
7 or 8 ice cubes
1 1/2 cups of soymilk

"I love the smell of Purple Smoothies in the morning. It Smells like Victory!"

This smoothie contains some beneficial blue, purple and black ingredients like blackberries, blueberries and blue preserve.

There are an unlimited number of variations for this smoothie because you can use different combinations of jams, preserves and fruits.

Maybe you also want to add some protein powder, organic ground flax seed, nuts or any other additional supplements that you prefer.

www.facebook.com/healthysmoothierecipes

You can also substitute the organic apple juice for the organic soymilk to make a tangier and more fruity blend.

This makes for the perfect breakfast smoothie to start your day in an energized and stress free way.

The Blackberry Blueberry Blue Preserve Energy Triangle Smoothie contains the following ingredients:

Ingredients:

1 1/2 cups of soymilk

3/4 cups of organic apple juice

1/2 cups plain bio or organic yogurt (I prefer to make my own home-made yogurts)

1 1/2 cups frozen blackberries

1/2 bag of frozen blueberries

2 tablespoons blueberry preserves

1 banana

ice cubes

www.facebook.com/healthysmoothiesrecipes

Directions:

For all these Smoothie recipe simply follow my 5 minute directions. Add all the ingredients into your Vitamix or similar high-speed blender.

Make sure to add fresh spring water if needed. Add as much water as you like in order to reach your desired thickness of the smoothie. For all the smoothie recipes, make sure to use organic products, fruits and vegetables if possible.

This is super easy to make. Just put all the ingredients into your high speed blender. Switch the blender to the highest level and blend until you do not hear any ice cubes crunching and until all ingredients are smooth.

Add more ice if needed and to your own liking.

You can adjust the raw organic honey to your preference or you can skip this step if you do not have a sweet tooth or if you are following a strict smoothie diet with unsweetened smoothies.

www.facebook.com/healthysmoothierecipes

Smoothie 14: The Coffee'n Cream Cinnamon Smoothie Booster

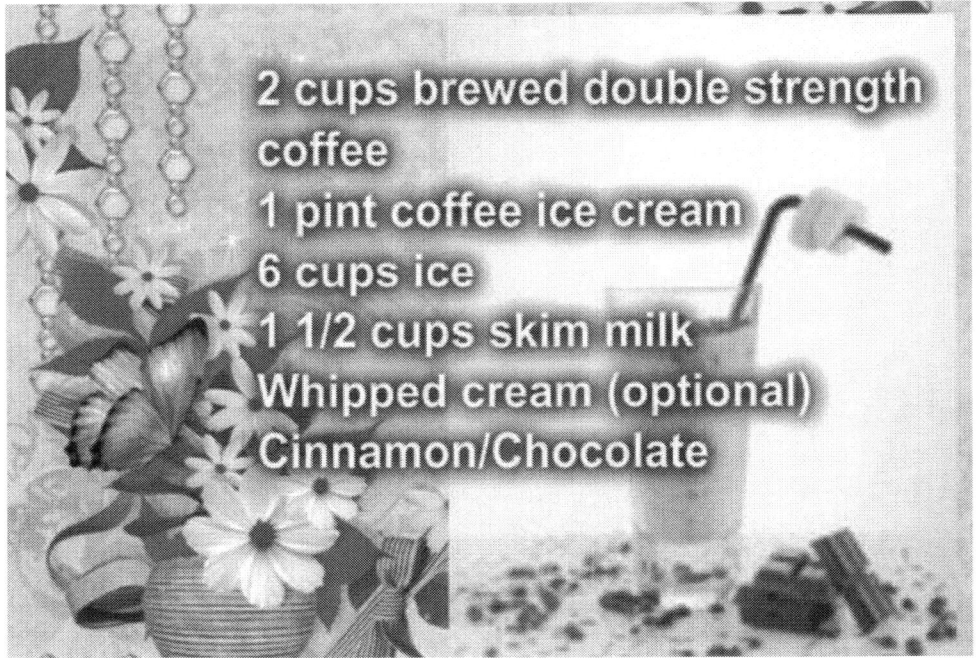

"I'm Going to Make him a Scrumptious Smoothie he can't Refuse."

The secret here is to enjoy the simple but effective blend of a rich tasting coffee in combination with the organic cinnamon and the taste of intelligence maker number one chocolate.

The Coffee'n Cream Cinnamon Smoothie contains the following ingredients:

www.facebook.com/healthysmoothiesrecipes

Ingredients:

2 cups of brewed double strength coffee (organic if possible)

1 pint of coffee ice cream (your favorite brand, I like mine organic)

1 1/2 cups of milk or skim milk

whipped organic cream (as a topping and if desired)

organic cinnamon and chocolate powder for the garnish

6 cups of ice cubes

Directions:

For all these Smoothie recipe simply follow my 5 minute directions. Add all the ingredients into your Vitamix or similar high-speed blender. Make sure to add fresh spring water or ice cubes if needed. Add as much water as you like in order to reach your desired thickness of the smoothie. For all the smoothie recipes, make sure to use organic products, fruits and vegetables if possible.

Mix all the ingredients together and process them with your favorite blender until all of the ingredients are well combined together. Make sure the broccoli is broken down and all the other ingredients are well swirled together in a rich looking creamy texture.

Blend the coffee, the ice cream, the ice cubes and the milk in your favorite high power blender. Mix everything until you get a smooth texture. Top the smoothie with some whipped cream and add some freshly grounded cinnamon and chocolate powder for the garnish.

www.facebook.com/healthysmoothierecipes

If you like you can also add some raw honey or if you are on a smoothie diet and like it sweet you can add a little bit of your favorite sweetener.

Other people love the unsweetened taste!

Smoothie 15: The Peanut Butter Banana Silk

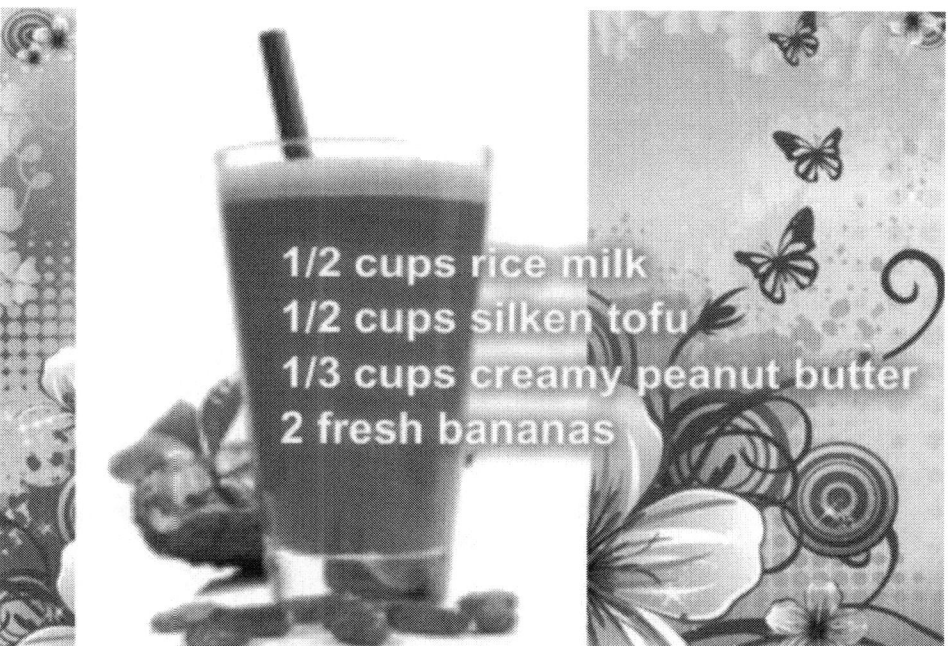

"All Great Things are Simple, and Many can be Expressed in Single Words: Freedom, Justice, Honor, Duty, Mercy, Hope, Smoothies."

Let's talk about this scrumptious peanut butter Banana Silk.

Peanuts are not only delicious but they are also very beneficial for the body and brain.

Peanuts are a rich source of antioxidants, they reduced risk of strokes, they help prevent gallstones, they protects against Alzheimer and other age related cognitive decline health problems.

www.facebook.com/healthysmoothierecipes

They are very rich in taste and the nutty flavor is popular amongst young and old. As opposed to people's opinion about nuts, they are in fact lowering the risk of weight gain.

The banana is a great combination with peanut butter as Elvis might confirm because he enjoyed his grand mother's and mother's peanut butter and banana sandwiches. He had too many in order to lose weight, but if you are respecting the ingredient list of this recipe, you are going to enjoy the health benefits of peanut butter in combination with bananas.

Here are some of the main health benefits of the banana. Bananas provide a very beneficial cardiovascular protection because of the potassium and fiber.

Bananas do sooth and protect from ulcers. They also improve elimination and protect your eyesight.

They help with your bones and they do promote kidney health.

The peanut butter Banana Silk Smoothie contains the following ingredients:

Ingredients:

1/2 cups of organic rice milk or hemp milk or coconut milk

1/2 cups of organic silken tofu

1/3 cups of creamy organic peanut butter

2 fresh organic bananas (sliced and frozen)

2 tablespoons of dark chocolate syrup

ice cubes

Directions:

For all these Smoothie recipe simply follow my 5 minute directions. Add all the ingredients into your Vitamix or similar high-speed blender. Make sure to add fresh spring water or ice cubes if needed. Add as much water as you like in order to reach your desired thickness of the smoothie. For all the smoothie recipes, make sure to use organic products, fruits and vegetables if possible.

Blend the organic rice milk, the tofu and the organic peanut butter in your favorite high speed blender. Add the banana frozen slices, the dark chocolate syrup and the ice cubes.

Blend on high speed until smooth, about 30 to 50 seconds.

Make sure the ingredients are broken down and all the other ingredients are well swirled together in a rich looking creamy and nutty texture.

Add a little more ice cubes if needed for your desired consistency.

If you like you can also add some raw honey or if you are on a smoothie diet and like it sweet you can add a little bit of your favorite sweetener.

Other people love the unsweetened taste!

www.facebook.com/healthysmoothierecipes

Smoothie 16: The Golden Delight

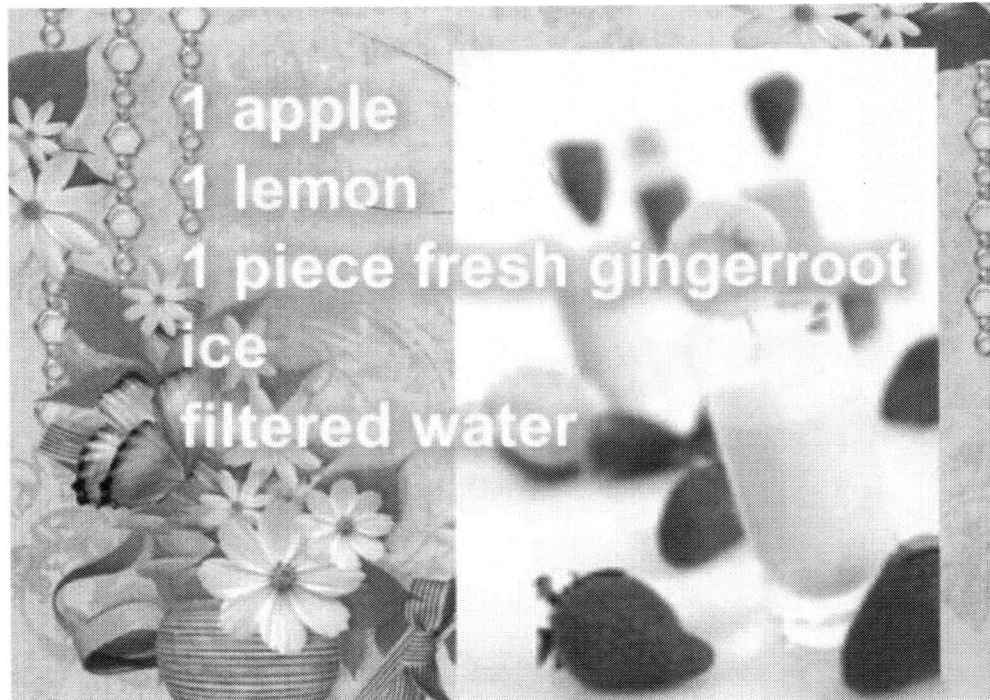

"We Are such Stuff As Golden Smoothies are Made of..."

Let's talk about a powerful combination of ginger root, lemon and apple.

The secret ingredient is the ginger root her and let's take a look at what the ginger root can do for you.

The anti inflammatory properties and active principles of the ginger root are thought to provide pain relief in multiple number of ways.

It has the power to stop migraines in their tracks and to ease the aches of arthritis and joint pain.

www.facebook.com/healthysmoothiesrecipes

It also fights ovarian cancer. It seems that ginger has the ability to eliminate the dangerous cancerous ovarian cells. Ginger also seems to slow the progress of bowel cancer.

Ginger also has a boosting effect on the immune system, making you fit and healthy.

Make sure to consume this immune system boosting smoothie drink on a daily basis to stay healthy and clean all year around!

I suggest to drink this smoothie in slow sips and you can keep it near your workspace so you can take a sip throughout the day. If you have trouble sleeping than make sure to only drink this secret ingredient drink in the morning because ginger has a similar characteristic as caffeine.

The peanut butter Banana Silk Smoothie contains the following ingredients:

Ingredients:

1 organic small apple (peeled, cored, sliced)

1 organic lemon (peeled, seeded)

1/2 cups of fresh filtered source water

ice cubes

1 piece of fresh gingerroot (peeled, crushed)

Directions:

For all these Smoothie recipe simply follow my 5 minute directions. Add all the ingredients into your Vitamix or similar high-speed blender.

www.facebook.com/healthysmoothierecipes

Make sure to add fresh spring water or ice cubes if needed. Add as much water as you like in order to reach your desired thickness of the smoothie. For all the smoothie recipes, make sure to use organic products, fruits and vegetables if possible.

Mix all the ingredients together and process them with your favorite blender until all of the ingredients are well combined together. Blend all ingredients together until smooth.

Make sure to drink the Golden Delight slowly.

Add a little filtered spring water or ice cubes if needed for your desired consistency.

If you like you can also add some raw honey or if you are on a smoothie diet and like it sweet you can add a little bit of your favorite sweetener.

Other people love the unsweetened taste!

Interactive Nutritious Ways

If you like to continue your path of learning more cool stuff about healthy living and healthy eating that will have an immediate effect on your life, you can do that via my interactive healthy nutrition system.

You can click the link below to download my interactive healthy nutrition learning device that you can use on your computer on a daily basis in order to live a healthier lifestyle!

My interactive healthy nutrition device it totally free for you because you bought this book, and I am always adding more value and more bonuses to this book in order to reward my customers and give them the most valuable and usable learning experience that I have tested out myself first and that will help you add more value, time and healthy quality of life to your lifestyle which is the goal of this system.

In order to get your own interactive healthy nutrition system on your own computer, you just have to download the program via the link below.

I am constantly adding more helpful and valuable healthy nutrition tips, ideas and ways to make your life healthier and thus more enjoyable to this

www.facebook.com/healthysmoothierecipes

program. It gets updated on a regular basis to reflect the latest proven and tested ways.

You will learn little valuable tidbits that make your body and mind healthier and life more enjoyable to live.

For example, did you know about these 10 foods that you absolutely must prevent?

I am using this knowledge every day to keep my life healthy, my food clean and my body and brain unharmed and I feel top fit and energized because of it.

This single action of preventing these types of foods is going to instantly add more energy to your body and you will feel less tired and stressed.

This result is huge and totally worth applying to your own daily nutrition ritual.

I will be sharing these kind of tips, hacks, and nuggets that will give you the results so that you can lead a happier, healthier, more successful, and more effective life!

Use my healthy nutrition system today and live a cleaner and healthier lifestyle and live more...
http://www.answerszone.info/Nutrition.exe

www.facebook.com/healthysmoothiesrecipes

Use my healthy nutrition system today and live!

www.facebook.com/healthysmoothierecipes

Blender Recipes For Weight Loss Quiz

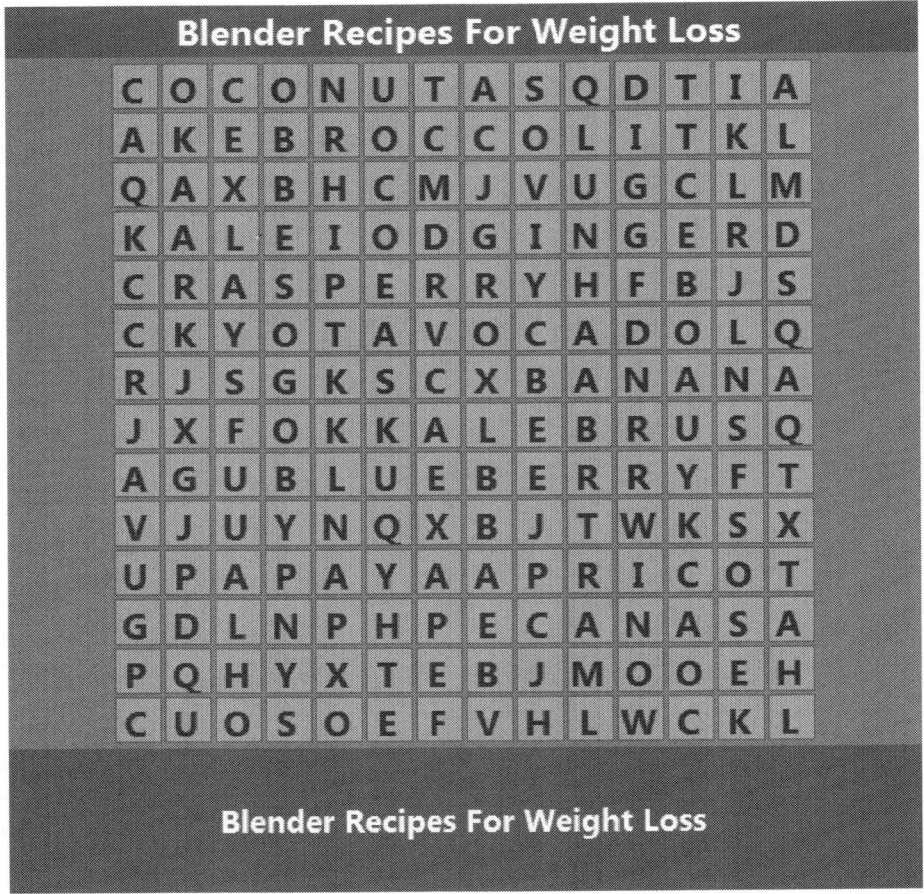

All you have to do is find 12 blender recipes for weight loss ingredients. Use your imagination, read backwards, sidewards, and forwards to find the correct words and associations. Go to the next page to see the correct answers! Have Fun!

www.facebook.com/healthysmoothiesrecipes

Notes

Answers

1. Avocado
2. Blueberry
3. Coconut
4. Ginger
5. Kale
6. Rasperry
7. Lemon
8. Papaya
9. Broccoli
10. Apricot
11. Banana
12. Pecan

www.facebook.com/healthysmoothiesrecipes

Conclusion

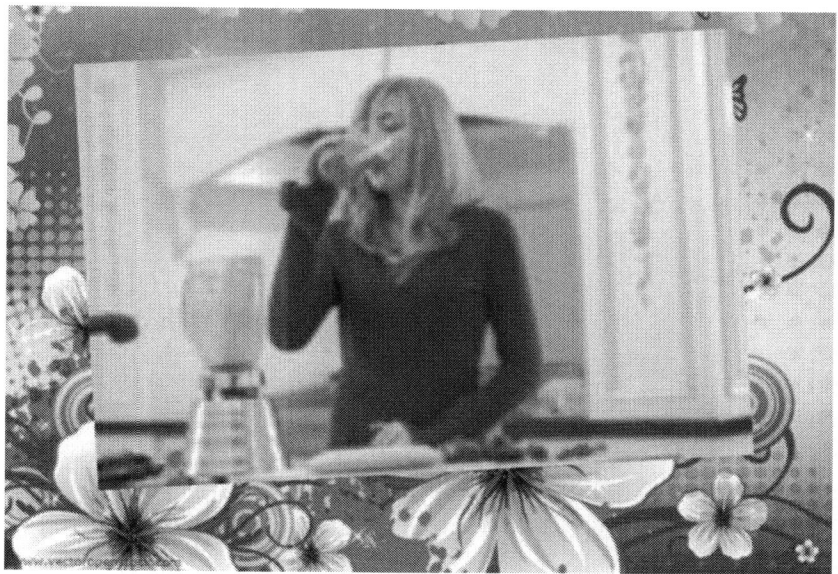

My goal with these high-speed blender recipes (in my case I am using the Nutribullet which is my favorite blender) is to give you some delicious blender recipes that are tasty in flavor and that will on the other hand help you with your weight loss goals.

These blender recipes for weight loss and detox are also 5 minute quick to make.

If you drink these nutritious and healthy 5 minute quick lean & clean drink recipes on a daily basis and add a daily workout plan like yoga or any other workout to your daily chores, you will take even more benefits out of your weight loss.

I love these recipes as they help me keep healthy, lean and satisfied.

www.facebook.com/healthysmoothierecipes

Each day I will use one or more of these wonderful recipes as a meal replacement for breakfast, lunch or dinner. The best part about using these different drinks is they actually work!

All of the ingredients that you need in order to make these recipes can be found at your local market for less than $9 which makes them affordable, too.

I hope I have delivered and fulfilled my promises and I hope that you are taking action on your own weight loss goals. If you do, you are going to be hooked on this smoothie diet for life!

I encourage you to take note of the many health benefits that come with each individual blender recipe's ingredients.

I also encourage you to take the book/device with you as you go and prepare each individual recipe.

Just keep the book on your mobile device next to your working table and go through one recipe at a time and as you progress. The book is intended to be used as a mental stimulation and to motivate you to take action at the same time.

I tried to make it as effortless, entertaining, inspirational and easy to use and consume as possible.

I hope you will use and consume the content whenever you want to lose some weight and detox your body.

If you really use it as it is intended to be used (use it as you go through the recipes and keep the book close during your preparation time!) it is a very powerful way of discovering the unlimited world of lean & clean high-speed blender smoothie recipes for weight loss!

Remember, all you have to do is open the book and start with the first recipe preparation that you like to get started with. Go through all of them and apply them on a daily basis as you see fit and depending on the health and weight loss benefits that you are looking to achieve.

You just need 5 minutes per preparation to be able to make at least one high-speed blender recipe per day. You can repeat the 5 minute quick preparation time as you see fit during your day.

For example, I am really big on Smoothies because they have helped me beat my Asthma in combination with a daily Yoga workout and therefore I am consuming at least 3 high-speed smoothies during the day when I am at home. It takes me not more than 15 minutes per day with the help of my beloved Nutribullet blender.

In addition to beating my health problems I was able to lose 40 lbs over the period of 2 month.

Everyone has a different goal, but these 5 minute quick and easy recipes that I have been able to perfect with the Nutribullet have certainly made my life easier, disease free, stress-free, cleaner & leaner.

Remember, you can achieve the maximum benefits (weight loss, health, detox, stress free lifestyle, and more) from consuming these high-speed blender (Nutribullet) recipes, too. In combination with a light workout these recipes really do wonderful things for your body and brain and weight loss will be an easy goal with these delicious tasting smoothies if you are going to take action on this!

Once you have achieved your own goal that you are looking to achieve with these amazing high-speed blender recipes by following these easy to follow instructions, you can go ahead

and discover even more of these healthy, lean & clean drink ingredients and what they can do for you.

www.facebook.com/healthysmoothierecipes

I believe with all the above high-speed blender recipes for weight loss & detox, you will become a lean, fit, healthy and energized person. These smoothies are going to help you become more productive in a stress free way, too.

I am already working on some more clean & lean high-speed blender recipes for you. Once I am done proving and testing them, I will release them as into this blender recipes series.

I will keep you updated on my new release if you like. To keep yourself updated, please visit my healthy smoothie recipe Facebook page here:
http://www.facebook.com/healthysmoothiesrecipes

Book 2 JUICING: Juicing For Vitality

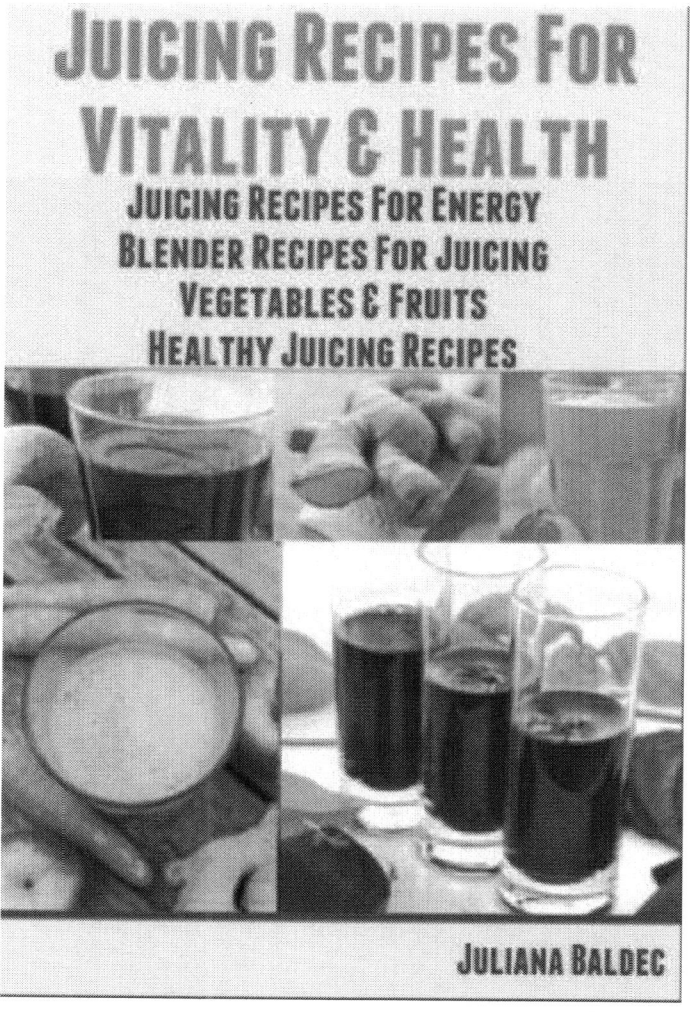

www.facebook.com/healthysmoothierecipes

My Favorite Quote

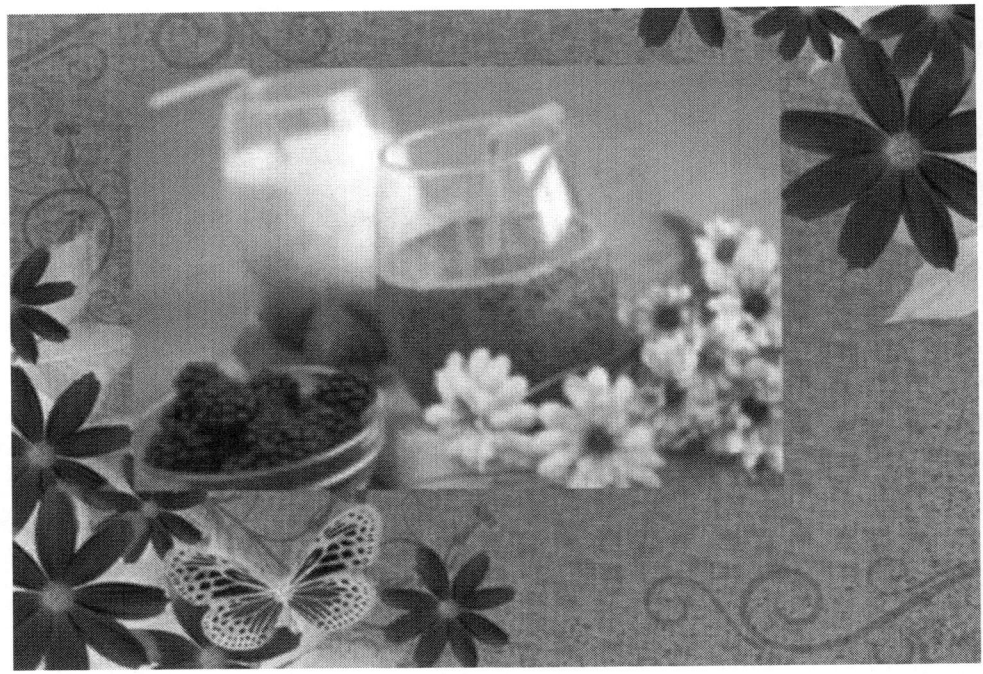

"Juices of fruits and vegetables are pure gifts from Mother Nature and the most natural way to heal your body and make yourself whole again." — Farnoosh Brock

www.facebook.com/healthysmoothiesrecipes

Why You Should Read This Book

Juicing is beneficial to your health, but what if you're looking to juice for a specific health benefit? Find and choose the benefit you're looking to juice for below!

Applying a daily juicing ritual will help with the following:

Vitality

Energy

Weight Loss (I lost 40 lbs by combining smoothies and juicing)

Natural Beauty & Skin Care

Protection & Healing

Antioxidants

Alzheimer's Prevention

Asthma Help (I suffered for years from breathing problems and Asthma and finally was able to get rid of it because of my daily Juicing and Smoothie ritual)

Blood Cleanse

Arthritis Prevention

Respiration & Asthma Relief

Bone Protection

www.facebook.com/healthysmoothierecipes

Cancer Prevention

Cervical Cancer Prevention

Breast Cancer Prevention

Colon Cancer Prevention

Liver Cancer Prevention

Lung Cancer Prevention

Prostate Cancer Prevention

Cataracts Prevention

Ovarian Cancer Prevention

Stomach Cancer Prevention

Digestion

Detoxification

Digestion

Heart Disease Prevention

Immune System

Hydration

Improving Eyesight

Improved Complexion

Increased Blood Circulation

Kidney Cleanse

Increased Libido

Liver Cleanse

Lower Blood Pressure

Lower Cholesterol

Macular Degeneration Prevention

Mental Health

Osteoporosis Prevention

Pain Relief

Reduce Inflammation

Reduce Water Retention

Stroke Prevention

More Benefits From Applying A Daily Juicing Habit:

Increase in energy and alertness as well as a renewed sense overall health and vigor

When you lean the art of juicing you can enjoy delicious and freshly made fruit and veggie juices to boost your system

Enjoy drinking morning boosting juices to get your day started and to be ready to face new challenges

www.facebook.com/healthysmoothierecipes

Play with all kinds of flavors and combinations of ingredients in order to find the one combination that you simply can not live without anymore

You can say no to sick making preservatives, chemicals, additives, and yes to natural sweeteners and a wonderful flavor experience

Discover all kinds of juices that you can make and use for other things like:

Freezing your own juices for later usage

Use your homemade juices for your own self-made cooking and baking recipes like pies, breads, soups, sauces, muffins, cakes and many other delicious treats

The juice makes an excellent stock or natural source of sweetener and they are much easier for the body to process than refined sugars

When you really put your mind to juicing, I imagine you will be amazed by all the wonderful uses you can find with these magical, healthy and healing juices

Welcome to the wonderful and magical world of juicing!

www.facebook.com/healthysmoothiesrecipes

Introduction

"The word juicing scares people because they think that drinking liquid is dieting. What they don't realize, is that they are regenerating their blood, cells, and organs to live a longer fulfulling life."

Welcome to the wonderful world of juicing!

Thank you for purchasing my juicing book that not only helped me in association with drinking smoothies to lose 40 lbs over two month, but I gained many other things from such a lifestyle change.

Since I have been changing my lifestyle to integrate juices in combination with smoothies into my lifestyle and since I have made a habit out of drinking juices and smoothies on a daily basis, I have been able to boost up my vitality, energy & health in general.

This is also the reason why I wrote a second book in my juicing book series. The first concentrates more on the aspect of juices in relation to weight loss and this second one is focused on juicing recipes for vitality, energy & health.

I am consuming my juices and smoothies on a daily basis and I have never been feeling more energized, stress free and fit.

I am going to share my positive health experiences with juicing in this book.

If your goal is to live a more healthy and clean lifestyle to double your life and boost up your health, these are the recipes that you should be consuming on a daily basis.

www.facebook.com/healthysmoothierecipes

Make sure to consume a combination of healthy smoothies and juices on a daily basis. This combination strategy is what helped me in the end become successful with my goal (increase my vitality and energy). Combining juices and smoothies also provides you with more different types of healthy drink variations which makes the whole process more fun and exciting.

You can also check out my Smoothies series at the end of this book in order to create your own collection of drink variations.

Just one last tip before we get started with the actual recipes.

These healthy ingredients and nutrients that are inside these juices do even become more beneficial to your body and mind if used and consumed in combination with a light yoga workout or any other workout that you prefer.

Before getting started with my daily juicing and smoothie ritual I had some serious health issues like breathing problems and asthma, stress and sleeping problems, but since I included daily Yoga combined with these healthy juices and smoothies, I am a new person.

Feeling sick is an experience of my past.

I am so happy that I got started with changing my lifestyle from a common and unhealthy meal plan to one that includes these delicious and healthy juices which kind of transformed my life into a balanced, healthy, energized and clean lifestyle!

I am enjoying this lifestyle so much that I decided to motivate and encourage others to get started with juicing for health benefits, too.

Depending on your own goals and preferences, you can either consume juices to become a healthier you or you can apply

www.facebook.com/healthysmoothiesrecipes

them as a juicing diet or a combination of juicing and smoothie diet in order to develop a leaner body or to lose some pounds. The first book in this series concentrates more on the weight loss aspects of juicing.

Make sure to first consult your doctor or physician to make sure that this diet is a good fit for your own personal situation.

Preparing these healthy juices with pulp does not take much time out of your schedule, and if you'd like to learn some cool time management tricks that apply to a healthy lifestyle that includes disciplines like yoga and/or meditation then I highly recommend my sister's book series that you can find on Amazon as well.

She calls it her Daily Ritual Yoga and Meditation Lifestyle series. You can check out her Yoga & Meditation lifeystle books by typing in her name: Alecandra Baldec into Amazon.com.

Each juicing recipe for weight loss includes a list of ingredients that you need to have in order to get started. Each healthy juice recipe does not take longer than 5 minute in terms of preparation.

For each juice recipe, simply follow my 5 Minute 6 Step Juicing System chapter and make sure to use organic products, fruits and vegetables whenever you can.

You can check out my smoothie books at the back of this book or by going to my full catalog of books. Just type in Juliana Baldec into Amazon.com and you will find all my books.

I hope you enjoy the book and I hope that you will get lots of inspiration and stimulation out of the book in order to be able to take advantage and be empowered by the fact that these healthy juices are helping you tap into some very powerful health benefits.

www.facebook.com/healthysmoothierecipes

Remember, each and every recipe and ingredient has its own health benefits!

All you have to do is identify your goal and take your daily action steps. If you follow my juicing for vitality and energy ritual from this book, you will have the same success with these delicious and healthy juices.

If you are looking to become healthier, make sure to integrate more and more of these juice recipes into your daily meal plan.

Everybody has a different goal and you can consume more or less of these juices depending on your personal situation, your goal and your
lifestyle.

One thing is for sure, if you get yourself into the habit of consuming these juices, you will empower and transform your body and mind with the result of a healthier, fitter, cleaner, more vital and more energized you!

www.facebook.com/healthysmoothiesrecipes

The 5 Minute 6 Step Juicing System

Step by Step Instructions For Juicing

For all these juicing recipe simply follow my 5 minute step by step instructions.

Step 1

Wash all veggies and fruits. Going through this thorough cleaning process will help prevent a nasty food-borne disease. I love to use organic vinegar because it is the most natural and organic solution, buy there are other options available if you prefer using products that are specifically designed for washing vegetables and fruits.

Step 2

Peel and cut all your fruits and veggies. Remember, you are juicing raw vegetables. This is why you need to cut them into small pieces before you get started. Especially if you are applying crunchier fruits and veggies such as carrots. Some high speed or high power juicers or a combination of juicer/blender like the Vitamix are able to take veggies and fruits in their whole form. In this case just follow the manufacturer's manual. Peel the skin of all your veggies and fruits. You also need to peel fruits like apples, melons, bananas, papaya, mango, pineapple, kiwis, banans, avocados, etc.

Next cut and chop the fruits and veggies such as leafy greens and fruits.

Step 3

Put your fruits and veggies into your favorite juicer or blender or a combination of juicer/blender (Nutribullet) and strictly follow the directions of the manual that comes with your machine. The manual will tell you what buttons to punch and what speed to use.

Juice the softer fruits/textures first.

You will see that when you are juicing the crunchier veggies and fruits they will help you push the softer and more delicate fruits and veggies through the blades.

If you are not using a juicer and only have a blender available, make sure to first strain the juice from citrus fruits like oranges, lemons, grapefruit, etc. When you are finished you can either leave the pulp inside the juice or take it out. It is totally up to your preference.

Next add the juice back to your mixture in the blender and proceed from there.

Step 4:

Juice and blend everything together as per instructions from your manual. You can always add some raw honey or sweetener depending on your goal with these juices. If the juice is too strong for you, you might also add some ice cubes or source water.

I only add ice cubes and water to smoothies, but some friends of mine who got started with juicing told me that some of the juices were too strong for them and they added ice cubes or water. In the summer time, ice cubes might be a refreshing alternative.

You will see that experimenting with your juicing process will help you discover many varieties and alternatives which makes juicing such a fun and exciting experience.

Step 5:

Try a variety of fruit and vegetable mixtures. As you experiment with juicing, you will find many combinations that you will enjoy on a daily basis.

www.facebook.com/healthysmoothiesrecipes

Some that pair well include apples with carrots, and leafy greens with kiwi. Try anything you want to taste. Create several go to recipes for yourself that you can use to make a healthy habit out of juicing.

Step 6:

The last step is a very important one if you want to enjoy your juicer/blender for a very long time.

Make sure to clean your machine ASAP and once you are done with your juice.

This helps prevent nasty bacteria growth and in order to prevent any diseases that related to hygiene.

Use warm water and dish soap. You can also use vinegar to clean and then run the pieces through the dishwasher.

If you do not have a dishwasher take extra care with the cleaning process.

Step 7:

Make sure to add lots of fiber to your smoothies, eat whole fruits and veggies throughout the day in order to stay balanced otherwise you might risk a dietary deficiency.

Step 8:
Enjoy your refreshing and delicious juice and get you day started with lots of vitality and energy...

Step 9:

Refer to chapter Juicing For Vitality & Energy to learn some more intriguing aspects that you can apply to your juicing lifestyle! The goal here is to keep the doctor away and reduce medical bills to ZERO cost and to double your life! (real money and time savers!)

www.facebook.com/healthysmoothierecipes

Notes

Why My Juicing Diet Works (My Secret Morning Elixir Ritual & Benefits)

With a consumption of these detoxing and healthy juicing recipes, I was finally able to reboot my system.

I am respecting my daily juicing ritual because it provides me with lots of energy and vitality. It is not hard anymore like it was when I first got started.

The secret to a healthy body with lots of energy and vitality is to get started with juicing and to apply this secret morning elexir on a daily basis.

Here is my secret lemon morning elixir that I drink every morning before I have my first juice.

Ingredients:

1 cup of warm or room temperature source water

Juice from 1 lemon (organic if possible)

1 teaspoon of raw apple cider vinegar

A pinch of cinnamon

1 teaspoon of raw honey (alternatively you can also use a couple drops of stevia)

For example, you can use stevia if you are on a yeast cleansing diet or low sugar diet.

www.facebook.com/healthysmoothierecipes

I drink this every morning, whether I am "feasting" or not, this is my morning coffee and I enjoy my morning elexir ritual!

What this morning elixir ritual does for you:

This morning elixir stimulates digestion and it releases toxins from the liver. It also jump starts your digestive enzymes.

Benefits of this morning lemon elixir ritual:

Raw honey benefits:

* Raw honey is loaded with minerals, vitamins & enzymes
* It helps cleanse your liver, flushes out fat from your body when done first thing in the morning on an empty stomach and remove toxins
* Raw honey soothes indigestion (it relieves acidity in your stomach)
* Energy booster
* Anti microbial and anti fungal
* Raw honey helps to keep your skin clear (it helps with skin conditions such as ring worms, eczema & psoriasis)

Apple Cider benefits:

* Apple Cider is a natural remedy for heartburn
* It can help clear up your skin conditions and acne
* It promotes digestion and apple cider will keep you regular
* Apple cider helps control weight
* It can help regulate your blood sugar

www.facebook.com/healthysmoothiesrecipes

* Apple Cider helps reduce sinus infections and sore throats

* It is very rich in potassium and enzymes

* It can help ease menstrual cramps

* It also helps promote youthful healthy bodies and skin

Lemon benefits:

* Lemon helps make the body more alkaline (increases pH)

* It provides lots of Vitamin C

* It purifies your blood and detoxes you

* Lemon is a cleansing agent & tonic for your liver by helping it produce more bile

Strawberry Carrot Beautifier

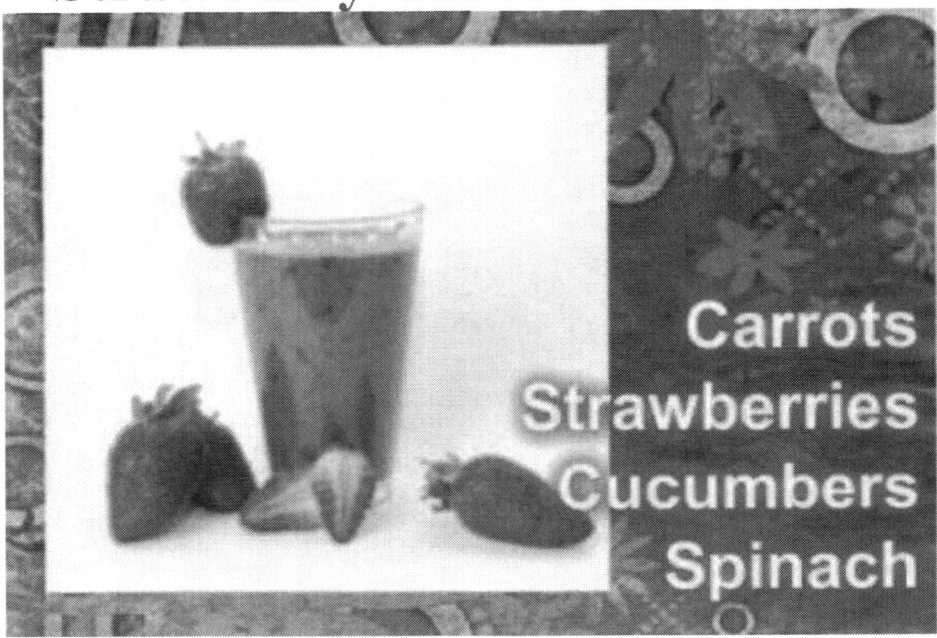

If developing your natural beauty is goal number one for you, this juice is a must! If you want to beautify yourself naturally, make sure to put the Strawberry Carrot Beautifier on your daily juice consumption list.

Pouring the contents of delightful strawberries and organic carrots or baby carrots into my favorite blender (in my case I am using the Nutribullet because it juices and keeps the pulp in the glass plus it also makes my favorite smoothies too) and whipping everything together into a zesty healthy natural beauty elixir is my second action every morning and I get my day started most of the times with this beauty drink. First I drink my Secret Morning Elixir and then I continue with my favorite drink that makes me beautiful in a natural way.

www.facebook.com/healthysmoothiesrecipes

This powerful beautifying Juice contains the following ingredients:

Ingredients:

8 medium to large organic carrots

10 strawberries (organic if possible)

3 cucumbers (organic if possible)

2 large handfuls of spinach (or baby spinach and organic if possible)

Directions:

For the directions please refer to the chapter where I am talking about my 5 Minute 6 Step Juicing System.

Here is a short instruction that sums up what to do. Make sure to refer back to my 6 step process for juicing so that you get the whole idea of juicing.

In this case peel the carrots and cucumbers.

Next cut and chop the washed fruits and veggies.

Put all the fruits and veggies from the ingredients list into your favorite juicer or blender or a combination of juicer/blender (Nutribullet) and strictly follow the directions of the manual that comes with your machine.

The manual of your favorite juicer/blender will tell you what buttons to push and what speed to use.

Juice the softer textures first.

www.facebook.com/healthysmoothierecipes

You will see that when you are juicing the crunchier veggies and fruits they will help you push the softer and more delicate fruits and veggies through the blades.

Juice and blend the all the ingredients together as per instructions.

You can always add some raw honey or sweetener depending on your goal with these juices. If the juice is too strong for you, you might also add some ice cubes or source water.

Enjoy your refreshing and delicious Powerful Strawberry Carrot Beautifier!

Lime Lemon Jalapeno Ginger Gold

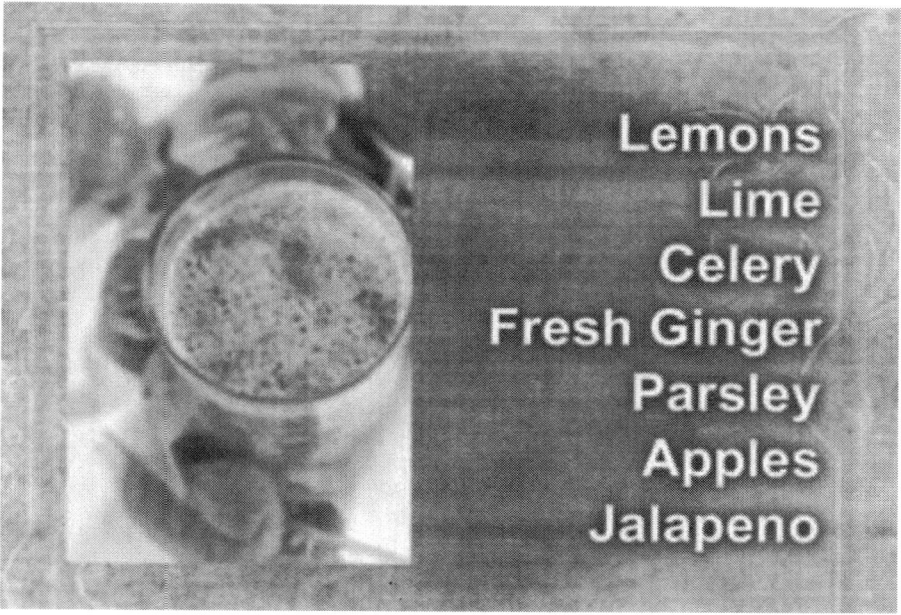

This is my favorite citrus tonic drink and I make sure to mix it into my daily meal plan because it helped me control my Asthma and breathing problems.

The secret combination of limes and lemons is what makes this juice a Vitamin C booster. It is a is also a great liver detoxifier.

In a condition of insufficient oxygen and breathing problems (mountain climbing, etc.) lemons are very helpful.

I suffered from Asthma and breathing problems and have been able to get rid of it by changing by eating and drinking habits. Drinking this juice is part of my daily juicing ritual.

www.facebook.com/healthysmoothierecipes

Vitamin C in lemons for example helps the body to neutralize free radicals that are linked to most types of diseases and aging.

The added health benefits of the ginger and the other ingredients are making this health elixir a vitality bomb!

This Lime Lemon Jalapeno Ginger Gold Elixir is a winner and it contains the following ingredients:

Ingredients:

2 Lemons with Skin and only if organic

1 Lime with skin and only if organic

10 Ribs of Celery (organic if possible)

2 inch of Fresh Ginger (organic if possible)

2 cups of Parsley (organic if possible)

2 Apples (any kind and organic if possible)

1/2 Jalapeno (this is a hot ingredient so be careful)

Alternative to the Jalapeno:

Sprinkle some cayenne pepper on top of your tonic drink when it's finished!

Directions:

For the directions please refer to the chapter where I am talking about my 5 Minute 6 Step Juicing System.

Here is a short instruction that sums up what to do. Make sure to refer back to my 6 step process for juicing so that you get the whole idea of juicing.

www.facebook.com/healthysmoothiesrecipes

In this case peel the ginger and the apples.

Next cut and chop the thoroughly washed veggies and fruits.

Put your ingredients into your favorite juicer or blender or a combination of juicer/blender (Nutribullet) and strictly follow the directions of the manual that comes with your machine.

Your blender manual will tell you what buttons to push and what speed to use.

Juice the softer textures first.

You will see that when you are juicing the crunchier veggies and fruits they will help you push the softer and more delicate fruits and veggies through the blades.

If you are not using a juicer and only have a blender available, make sure to first strain the juice from the lime and lemons.

Once it is finished you can either leave the pulp inside or take it out. This is totally up to your preference.

In this case you have to add the juices back to the blender and proceed from there.

Juice and blend the juice with the rest of your ingredients together as per instructions.

You can always add some raw honey or sweetener depending on your goal with these juices. If the juice is too strong for you, you might also add some ice cubes or source water.

Enjoy this Vitamin C enriched delicious tonic!

www.facebook.com/healthysmoothierecipes

www.facebook.com/healthysmoothiesrecipes

Grapefruit Cranberry Double Immune System Blaster

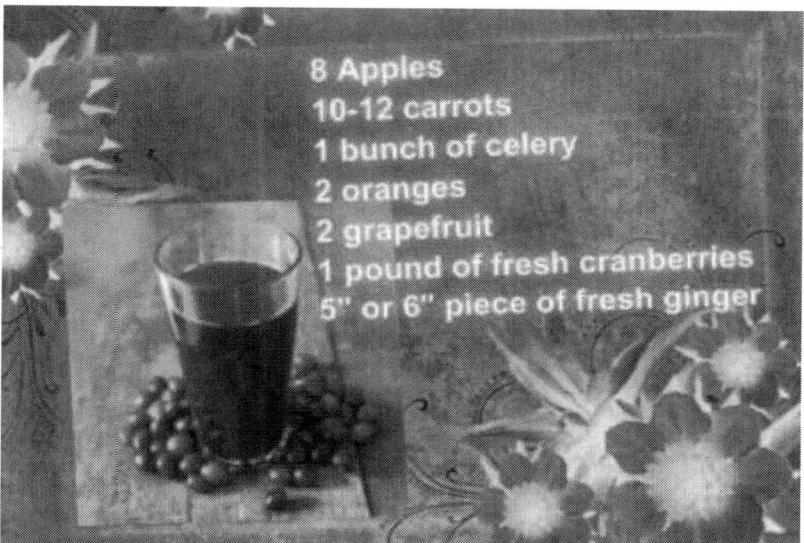

8 Apples
10-12 carrots
1 bunch of celery
2 oranges
2 grapefruit
1 pound of fresh cranberries
5" or 6" piece of fresh ginger

A combination of healthy superfood type of ingredients: cranberries and ginger is what this smoothie is all about. The Grapefruit Cranberry Double Immune System Blaster is a perfect solution if your goal is to follow a healthy and clean juicing lifestyle.

So what is so beneficial about juicing cranberries? Consuming cranberries in their natural form (not buying cranberry juices with added sugar) has the following health benefits:

Cranberries are a protection against Urinary Tract Infection (UTI), they give anti-inflammatory benefits, cardiovascular benefits, antioxidant protection,
as well as anti-cancer benefits.

The intake of cranberry extracts has shown the ability to improve multiple aspects of immune functions and it has shown the ability to lower the frequency of cold and flu symptoms.

www.facebook.com/healthysmoothierecipes

Cranberries in combination with ingredients like ginger are even more powerful.

What makes the ginger so powerful in terms of health benefits?

The anti-inflammatory properties and active principles of the ginger root are thought to provide pain relief in multiple number of ways. It has the power to stop migraines in their tracks and to ease the aches of arthritis and joint pain.

It also fights ovarian cancer. It seems that ginger has the ability to eliminate the dangerous cancerous ovarian cells. Ginger also seems to slow the progress of bowel cancer.

Ginger also has a boosting effect on the immune system, making you fit and healthy.

Make sure to consume this immune system boosting smoothie drink on a daily basis to stay healthy and clean all year around!

I suggest to drink this juice in slow sips and you can keep it near your workspace so you can take a sip throughout the day.

Ginger also improves your breath. It can cleanse the palate leaving your mouth feeling refreshed.

Ginger protects against nuclear radiation and if you want to get the full benefits of this advantage you will have to consume a daily dose.

Ginger also strengthens your immunity. An improved immune system can mean that you get ill less often. It means that you will recover quicker. It also means that when everyone else around you is coming down with something you can stay fit and healthy.

Ginger also fights cancers. Ginger has been shown to help treat various forms of cancer, including ovarian cancer.
Ginger protects against Alzheimer's disease.

www.facebook.com/healthysmoothiesrecipes

Ginger helps to slow down the loss of brain cells that typically is the precursor to Alzheimer's disease.

Ginger is perfect for weight loss because it stimulates the appetite. If you have a very sluggish digestive system and find out that you need to get your digestive fire going before eating a meal, ginger can help you out.

Ginger can also help as an appetite stimulant to get your digestive juices flowing so that you are better able to digest foods and lose weight as a side effect because improper digestion of food leaves the food fermenting in your digestive system which can lead to weight gain as a side effect.

Ginger is a fat burning superfood and it acts as a fat burner. Ginger helps you feel satisfied and full. This means that you will eat less food which will help reducing your overall caloric intake in the end.

Ginger is a true magical secret ingredient and this juice combines ginger and turns it into an even healthier raw power cocktail.
I am enjoying the benefits of ginger every day. If I do not have enough time to make a juice because I am pressed in time, I consume at least a glass of ginger water or ginger tea with lemon.

If you are looking to lose weight like I did, you make sure to drink a glass of this magical ginger water or ginger/lemon water (cold or hot as herbal tea) throughout the day and in little sips. If you apply this ginger water method you will always feel full and satisfied.

I have tested this juice with a lot of friends and family members before adding it to my favorite collection of juices. They all got some great benefits out of drinking this health elixir on a daily basis.

www.facebook.com/healthysmoothierecipes

I am constantly testing and proving new juicing recipes that I am gradually adding to my "Tested & Proven Juicing Recipe Collection"

This one has passed the test because it is not only delicious, but it is such a healthy treat.

Celery might not sound appealing to you at first, but the combination of all the ingredients is turning this juice into an absolute winner. It does not only taste deliciously, but it provides your body and brain with a powerful mix of rejuvenating and healing nutrition.

This healthy elixir called the Grapefruit Cranberry Double Immune System Blaster contains the following ingredients:

Ingredients:

8 Apples (organic if possible)

10-12 carrots or baby carrots (organic if possible)

1 bunch of celery (organic if possible)

2 oranges (for juicing and organic if possible)

2 grapefruit (organic if possible)

1 pound of fresh cranberries (frozen are ok if you can't find fresh ones and organic if possible)

5" or 6" piece of fresh ginger (organic if possible)

Alternative Fruits:

You can also add pears, melons, grapes, whatever the season and whatever your taste is!

Directions:

For the directions please refer to the chapter where I am talking about my 5 Minute 6 Step Juicing System.

Here is a short instruction that sums up what to do. Make sure to refer back to my 6 step process for juicing so that you get the whole idea of juicing.

In this case peel the apples, carrots oranges, grapefruits and ginger.

Next cut and chop the fruits and veggies.

Put all the fruits and veggies from the ingredients list into your favorite juicer or blender or a combination of juicer/blender (Nutribullet) and strictly follow the directions of the manual that comes with your machine.

Your blender manual will tell you what buttons to push and what speed to use.

Juice the softer textures first.

You will see that when you are juicing the crunchier veggies and fruits they will help you push the softer and more delicate fruits and veggies through the blades.

If you are not using a juicer and only have a blender available, make sure to first strain the juice from the oranges and the grapefruits first.

Once it is finished you can either leave the pulp inside or take it out. This is totally up to your preference.

In this case you have to add the juice back to the blender and proceed from there.

Juice and blend the juice with all the other ingredients together as per instructions.

www.facebook.com/healthysmoothierecipes

You can always add some raw honey or sweetener depending on your goal with these juices. If the juice is too strong for you, you might also add some ice cubes or source water.

Enjoy your refreshing and delicious Grapefruit Cranberry Double Immune System Blaster!

Liquid Tomatoe Booster

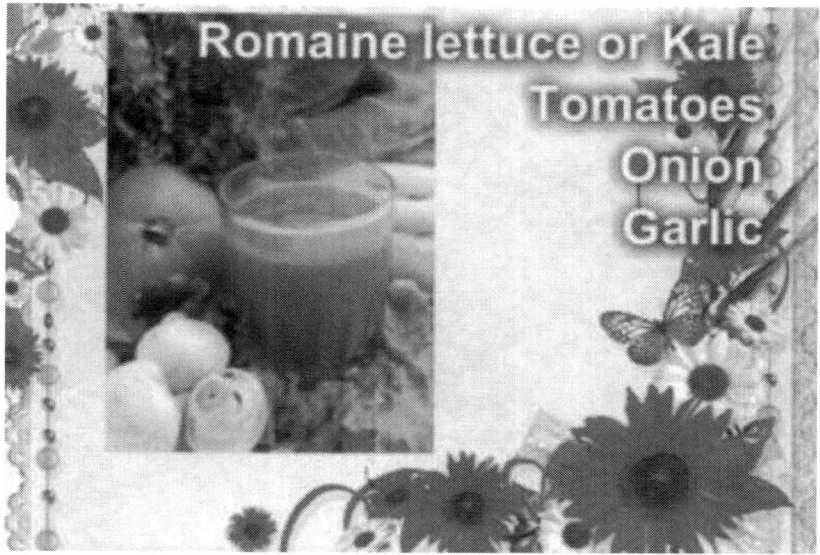

This is another one of my natural beauty juices. I make sure to mix it at least 3 to 4 times into my weekly meal plan because I enjoy the beautifying benefits of it. It really makes my skin soft, hydrated and wrinkle free. I apply some powerful organic and self made beauty products to my skin (cocoa butter, apple cider, honey and aloe) and like this (juicing + natural self made beauty products) my body is able to stay beautiful from the inside out.

I am working on a new series where I divulge my organic homemade skin care and beauty secrets and you can soon check it out and add these beauty secrets to your own home spa and beauty program, too.

A combination of juices and smoothies, the benefits from my self made beauty and skin care system and a light yoga and meditation workout is all I need in order to create the ultimate healthy lifestyle for myself and my family.

This red beauty juice is a fortified and nutritious combination of vitality boosting superfood reds and greens like tomatoes, kale, lettuce, swiss chard, and romaine.

Mixing nutritious veggies and greens like tomatoes, onions, garlic, kale and all types of different salads will bring an almost sweet taste to this juice because the tomato fruits (yes tomatoes are fruits!) help neutralize strong and bitter flavours that might come from the veggies and greens.

The ginger gives this juice drink some powerful health benefits like immune boosting actions.

The reason kale is becoming popular is because it helps you fill up without a lot of calories to speak of. It doesn't have any fat, has plenty of fiber as well as iron and Vitamin K. Because of its antioxidant content you'll get anti-inflammatory benefits which helps to reduce the symptoms of inflammation, while also helping to avoid the rise of certain diseases. It also helps to restore and maintain an alkaline state.

This Liquid Tomato Booster contains the following ingredients:

Ingredients:

1 bunch of Romaine lettuce (organic if possible)

6 medium ripe tomatoes (organic if possible)

1 thick slice of Vidalia or other mild onion (about 1/4" thick and organic if possible)

5-6 cloves fresh, peeled garlic (organic if possible)

You can substitute Swiss Chard or Kale for the Romaine (organic if possible)

5" or 6" piece of fresh ginger (organic if possible)

Directions:

For all these For the directions please refer to the chapter where I am talking about my 5 Minute 6 Step Juicing System.

Here is a short instruction that sums up what to do. Make sure to refer back to my 6 step process for juicing so that you get the whole idea of juicing.

In this case peel the tomatoes, the onion, the ginger and the garlic.

Next cut and chop the fruits and veggies.

Put all the fruits and veggies from the ingredients list into your favorite juicer or blender or a combination of juicer/blender (Nutribullet) and strictly follow the directions of the manual that comes with your machine.

Your blender manual will tell you what buttons to push and what speed to use.

Juice the softer textures first.

You will see that when you are juicing the crunchier veggies they will help you push the softer and more delicate veggies through the blades.

Juice and blend all the ingredients from the list above together as per instructions.

If the juice is too strong for you, you might also add some ice cubes or source water.

Enjoy your refreshing Liquid Tomato Booster that will beautify and energize you from the inside out!

www.facebook.com/healthysmoothierecipes

Double Melon Elexir

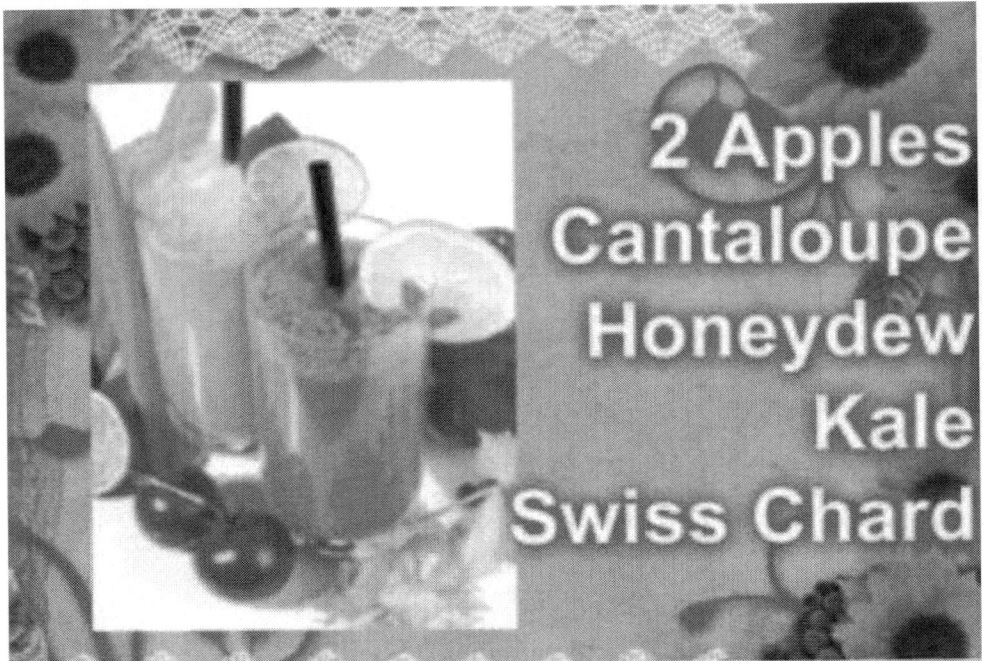

If you love tasty juices with some powerful orange and green ingredients that are super healthy and taste deliciously, then you might consider the Double Melon Elixir.

Cantaloupes are a rich source of folates, carotenoids, potassium, and vitamin C.

They grow naturally in Africa and Asia. People eat cantaloupes because of its juicy, tasty flavor. Some people even use it as an appetizer and as an ingredient for salads.

Honeydews are rich in potassium, vitamin C, copper, B vitamins.

One cup of honeydew will provide about half of your daily vitamin C needs. Vitamin C helps boost your immune system which in turn will help prevent infections and illnesses.

www.facebook.com/healthysmoothiesrecipes

Honeydew melons are a member of the melon fruit family. Honeydew melon has pale green juicy and sweet flesh. Honeydew melons are a very nutritious addition for people who are on a diet. Honeydew melons also contain several vitamins and minerals. They only have 60 calories per half cup which makes them a very nutritionally beneficial fruit.

Pouring the contents of a delightful cantaloupe, honeydew, fresh apples, kale and swiss chard into your favorite blender (in my case I am using the Nutribullet because I love its flexibility) and whip it all together into a zesty nutritious rich elixir that heals from the inside out and keeps your body healthy and fit.

This sweet and tasty double melon elixir contains the following ingredients:

Ingredients:

2 Apples (organic if possible)

1/2 Cantaloupe (organic if possible)

1/2 Honeydew (organic if possible)

6-8 leaves Kale (organic if possible)

6-8 leaves Swiss Chard (organic if possible)

Directions:

For the directions please refer to the chapter where I am talking about my 5 Minute 6 Step Juicing System.

Here is a short instruction that sums up what to do. Make sure to refer back to my 6 step process for juicing so that you get the whole idea of juicing.

www.facebook.com/healthysmoothierecipes

In this case peel the apples and scrape out the juicy contents of the melons.

Next cut and chop the fruits and veggies.

Put all the fruits and veggies from the ingredients list into your favorite juicer or blender or a combination of juicer/blender (Nutribullet) and strictly follow the directions of the manual that comes with your machine.

The manual will tell you what buttons to push and what speed to use.

Juice the softer textures first.

You will see that when you are juicing the crunchier veggies and fruits they will help you push the softer and more delicate fruits and veggies through the blades.

Juice and blend all the ingredients from the list above together as per instructions.

You can always add some raw honey or sweetener depending on your goal with these juices. If the juice is too strong for you, you might also add some ice cubes or source water.

Enjoy this refreshing and hydrating Double Melon Health Elixir that will beautify and heal you from the inside out!

Zesty Blackberry Ginger Booster

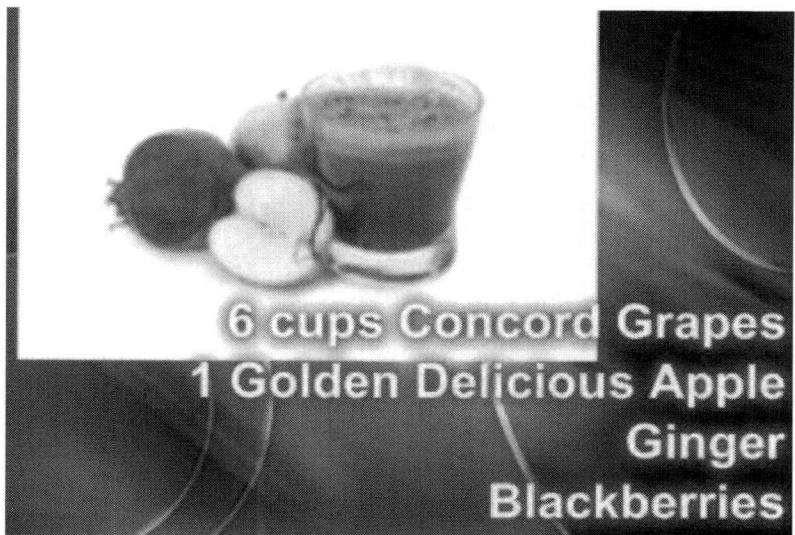

This is a fortified and nutritious combination of healthy and vitality boosting fruits such as grapes and blackberries.

This juice gets its rich flavour from the mix of this powerful combination of fruits.

This dark superfood cocktail also contains the benefits of zesty ginger that is swirled into the juice.

This juice makes for a perfect wholesome and healthy start of your day with lots of energy and vitality.

If you feel that the juice is too strong or too bitter, you can always add another sweet and juicy apple into the blend to make it sweeter in taste.

I enjoy this juice with the contents of at least 2 apples as a breakfast juice and I only use 1 apple if I consume this juice as a lunch or dinner juice. Usually I consume this recipe with only 1 apple instead of coffee after a light lunch meal.

The Zesty Blackberry Ginger Booster contains the following ingredients:

Ingredients:

6 cups of Concord Grapes (any grapes will do and organic if possible)

1 Golden Delicious Apple (organic if possible)

2" piece Ginger (organic if possible)

1/2 cup of Blackberries (organic if possible)

Directions:

For the directions please refer to the chapter where I am talking about my 5 Minute 6 Step Juicing System.

Here is a short instruction that sums up what to do. Make sure to refer back to my 6 step process for juicing so that you get the whole idea of juicing.

In this case peel the apple and ginger.

Next cut and chop the fruits.

Put all the fruits from the ingredients list into your favorite juicer or blender or a combination of juicer/blender (Nutribullet) and strictly follow the directions of the manual that comes with your machine.

Your juicer or blander manual will tell you what buttons to push and what speed to use.

Juice the softer textures first.

www.facebook.com/healthysmoothiesrecipes

You will see that when you are juicing the crunchier fruits they will help you push the softer and more delicate fruits through the blades.

Juice and blend the juices with the other ingredients from the list above together as per instructions.

You can always add some raw honey or sweetener depending on your goal with these juices. If the juice is too strong for you, you might also add some ice cubes or source water.

Enjoy this Blackberry Ginger Tonic and boost your body's vitality!

www.facebook.com/healthysmoothierecipes

Blueberry Coconut Veggie Detoxer

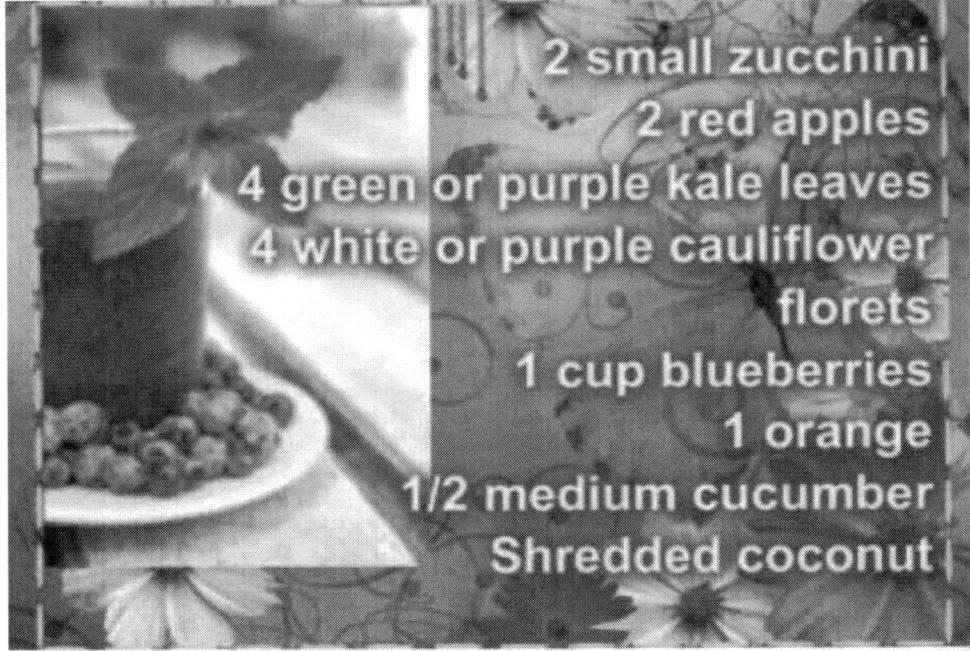

2 small zucchini
2 red apples
4 green or purple kale leaves
4 white or purple cauliflower florets
1 cup blueberries
1 orange
1/2 medium cucumber
Shredded coconut

Who says that vegetables are for lunch and dinner only? This leafy green cocktail contains delicious and zesty fruits that are swirled into the greens and this juice makes for a perfect wholesome and healthy start of your day so that you do not need to wait for lunchtime to eat these healthy veggies.

It does not only taste deliciously, but kale provides the body with anti inflammatory health benefits. The Vitamin C of the lemon detoxifies your body and destroys intestinal worms and the cauliflower

There are several dozen studies linking cauliflower containing diets to bladder cancer, breast cancer, colon cancer, prostate cancer, and ovarian cancer prevention.

www.facebook.com/healthysmoothiesrecipes

Cauliflower provides special nutrient support for the detox system, the antioxidant, and the inflammatory/anti-inflammatory system that are connected with cancer prevention and cancer development.

Chronic imbalances in any of these 2 systems of the body can increase the risk of cancer. When imbalances in all of the three systems occur simultaneously, the risk of cancer does increases significantly.

Cauliflower does provide the following health benefits. It gives detox support. It provides the body with antioxidant benefits, it provides ant-inflammatory benefits, it provides the body with cardiovascular support and digestive support.

The zucchini is one of the very low calorie vegetables because it only has 17 calories per 100 g. The zucchini contains no saturated fats or cholesterol. It is a good source of dietary fibers that do help reduce constipation which in turn offers some protection against colon cancer.

Zucchinis have an anti-oxidant value of around 180 Trolex Equivalents (TE) per 100g which is far below some of the superfood berries and vegetables. Nonetheless, the Zucchinis, especially golden skin zucchini varieties, are very rich in flavonoid poly-phenolic antioxidants such as lutein, carotenes, and zea-xanthin. These compounds do help scavenge harmful oxygen-derived free radicals. These compounds also do reactive oxygen species from the body that do play a critical role in the aging process and various other disease processes.

Courgettes which is another word for zucchinis also do have a relative moderate source of folates. Folates are important in cell division and the DNA synthesis. When taken in adequately before a pregnancy, zucchinis can help prevent neural tube defects in the unborn baby.

It is also a very rich source of potassium which is an important intra-cellular electrolyte. Potassium is also a very heart friendly electrolyte and it helps bring the reduction in blood pressure and heart rates.

Fresh zucchinis, indeed, are a rich source of anti oxidant vitamin C.

In addition, zucchinis contain moderate levels of B-complex groups of vitamins like pyridoxine, thiamin, riboflavin as well as minerals like manganese, iron, zinc, and phosphorus.

The coconut is the last secret ingredient of this elexir because the coconut oil that is contained in the coconut is highly beneficial for the health and beauty.

The coconut helps prevent obesity and it improves the heart health. It is high in dietary fiber.

Coconut fiber also slows down the release of glucose and it therefore requires less insulin to utilize the glucose and transports it into the cell. In the cell it is converted into energy.

Coconut assists in relieving stress on the pancreas and enzyme systems of the body. This in turn reduces the risk that is associated with Diabetes.

Coconut reduces sweet cravings and does improve the insulin secretion and the utilization of blood glucose.

The healthy fat in coconut slows down any rise in blood sugar.

The coconut improves digestion and many of the symptoms and inflammatory conditions associated with digestive and bowel disorders.

www.facebook.com/healthysmoothiesrecipes

It is a quick energy boost and provides your body with a quick energy boost - a super nutritious source of extra energy. Coconut is actually utilized by the body to produce energy, instead of storing it as body fat.

Coconut provides endurance during an athletic or physical performance. It promotes healthy thyroid functions.

Finally, coconut helps to relieve the symptoms of a chronic fatigue and vitalizes the body with a quick energy boost!

If you like the taste of coconut, I highly recommend to keep a glass of fresh coconut water next to you. This keeps you energized during the day in a very natural way!

The highly nutritious Blueberry Coconut Veggie Detoxer contains the following ingredients:

Ingredients:

2 small zucchini (organic if possible)

2 red apples (organic if possible)

4 green kale leaves (organic if possible)

4 white or purple cauliflower florets (organic if possible)

1 1/2 cup blueberries (organic if possible)

1 orange, peeled (use oranges that are best for juicing and never juice citrus fruits with the skin)

1 lemon (peeled and organic if possible)

1/2 medium cucumber (organic if possible)

Shredded coconut (only fresh and for added sweetness and totally optional)

www.facebook.com/healthysmoothierecipes

Directions:

For all these juice recipe For the directions please refer to the chapter where I am talking about my 5 Minute 6 Step Juicing System.

Here is a short instruction that sums up what to do. Make sure to refer back to my 6 step process for juicing so that you get the whole idea of juicing.

In this case peel the apples, orange, lemon, and cucumber.

Next cut and chop the fruits and veggies.

Put all the fruits and veggies from the ingredients list into your favorite juicer or blender or a combination of juicer/blender (Nutribullet) and strictly follow the directions of the manual that comes with your machine.

The manual will tell you what buttons to push and what speed to use.

Juice the softer textures first.

You will see that when you are juicing the crunchier veggies and fruits they will help you push the softer and more delicate fruits and veggies through the blades.

If you are not using a juicer and only have a blender available, make sure to first strain the juice from the orange and lemon.

Once it is finished you can either leave the pulp inside or take it out. This is totally up to your preference.

In this case you have to add the juice back to the blender and proceed from there.

www.facebook.com/healthysmoothiesrecipes

Juice and blend the juices with the other ingredients from the list above together as per instructions.

You can always add some raw honey or sweetener depending on your goal with these juices. If the juice is too strong for you, you might also add some ice cubes or source water.

Enjoy this powerful and tasty Blueberry Coconut Veggie Detoxer!

Orange Breakfast Power Cocktail

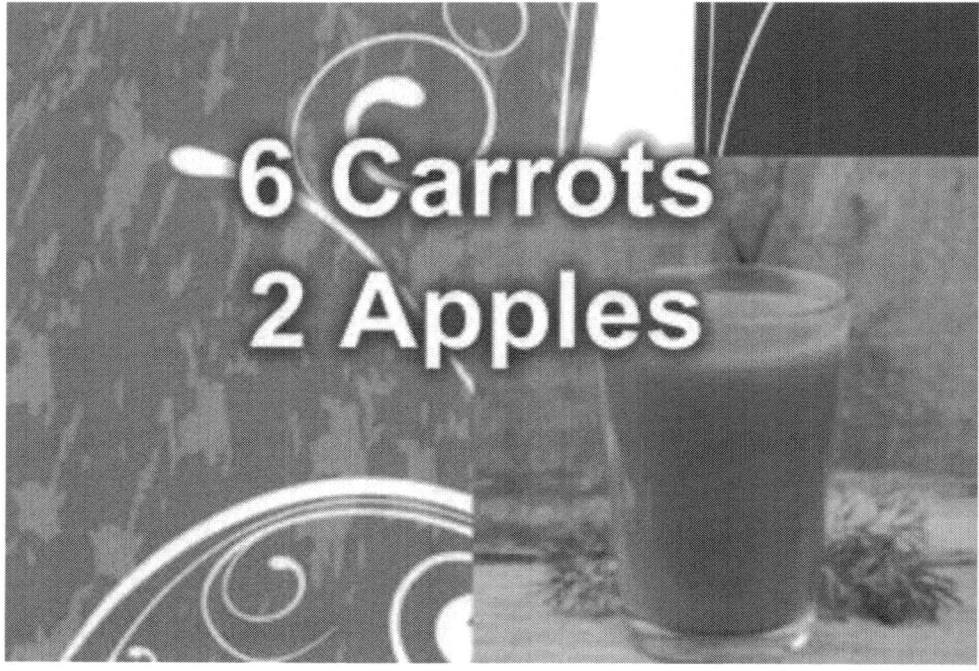

"Oranges strengthen your emotional body, encouraging a general feeling of joy, well-being, and cheerfulness." - Tae Yun Kim

Let's talk about this simple and yet powerful combination of apples and carrots. The secret of this juice lies in its simplicity.

Let's take a look at what an apple a day can do for you in combination with carrots.

Carrots have lots of health benefits. Carrots help improve the eye visions because carrots are rich in beta-carotene. Beta-

Carotene is converted into vitamin A in the liver. Vitamin A is then transformed in the retina.

Some other health benefits are cancer prevention, anti-aging, healthy glowing skin, prevention from infections, beautiful and rejuvenated skin, prevention from heart disease, body cleansing, healthy teeth and gums, and stroke prevention.

Medical studies have shown that carrots help reduce the risk of breast cancer, lung cancer, and colon cancer. Researchers have just discovered falcarindiol and falcarinol which cause the anticancer properties.

The high level of beta carotene acts as an antioxidant to cell damage that is done to the body through regular metabolism. Carrots help slow down the aging of the cells.

Carrots are known to prevent infection. If you cut yourself, try shredded raw or boiled mashed carrots as a natural solution to prevent infections.

Diets that contain a high amount of carotenoids are associated with a lower risk of heart diseases. A regular consumption of carrots also helps minimize the cholesterol levels. The soluble fibers contained in these delicious and crunchy carrots bind with bile acids.

Vitamin A helps the liver in flushing out toxins and waste from the body. It reduces the bile and the fat in the liver. The fibers that are present in the carrots do help clean out the colon.

Crunchy carrots also help clean your mouth and teeth. Carrots scrape off plaque and food particles in a natural way. Carrots stimulate gums and trigger a lot of saliva. The minerals in carrots prevent tooth damage, too.

Crunching carrots or juicing carrots will also help protect against strokes.

Mixing carrot juice together with orange juice becomes even more powerful.

www.facebook.com/healthysmoothierecipes

Here is what oranges can do for you. Oranges are nutritional and powerful fruits because they provide an array of health benefits to your body. Oranges have a wealth of nutrients including vitamin A precursors, vitamin C, calcium, potassium, and pectin.

Oranges alkalize the body, protect your skin, help with the regulation of a high blood pressure in the body, help create good eye vision, and relieve constipation.

They are also very effective in fighting against viral infections.

Oranges are very rich in citrus limonoids, which is proven to help fight a number of varieties of cancers, including skin cancer, stomach cancer, lung cancer, breast cancer, stomach cancer, and colon cancer.

They are very effective in fighting against viral infections.

Drinking orange juice regularly reduces the risk of kidney stones and prevents kidney diseases.

Since oranges are full of soluble fiber, oranges are helpful in lowering the cholesterol level. Oranges are also full of potassium, an electrolyte mineral that is responsible for helping the heart function. When these potassium levels go down, you may develop an abnormal heart rhythm.

Lastly, oranges are full of vitamin C which protects your cells by neutralizing free radicals. Free radicals do cause chronic diseases, like heart diseases and cancer.

As you can see carrots and oranges provide lots of powerful health benefit and they taste deliciously, too, and who does not like to enjoy a juicy orange snack or drink or like to crunch tasty carrots with healthy dips

Oranges are very popular with athletes because oranges can be easily taken in for a quick burst of energy.

www.facebook.com/healthysmoothiesrecipes

Apart from drinking this orange carrot juice on a daily basis, I also love eating one or two oranges a day and for that same energy-boosting effects as athletes are doing it.

This Orange Breakfast Power Cocktail contains the following ingredients:

Ingredients:

6 carrots (organic if possible)
2 apples (organic if possible)

Directions:

For all these juice recipe For the directions please refer to the chapter where I am talking about my 5 Minute 6 Step Juicing System.

Here is a short instruction that sums up what to do. Make sure to refer back to my 6 step process for juicing so that you get the whole idea of juicing.

In this case peel the apples and carrots.

Next cut and chop them up.

Put them into your favorite juicer or blender or a combination of juicer/blender (Nutribullet) and strictly follow the directions of the manual that comes with your machine.

The manual will tell you what buttons to punch and what speed to use.

Juice and blend them together as per instructions of your machine's manual.

www.facebook.com/healthysmoothierecipes

You can always add some raw honey or sweetener depending on your goal with these juices. If the juice is too strong for you, you might also add some ice cubes or source water.

Enjoy this Orange Breakfast Power Cocktail!

www.facebook.com/healthysmoothiesrecipes

Full Body Detoxer

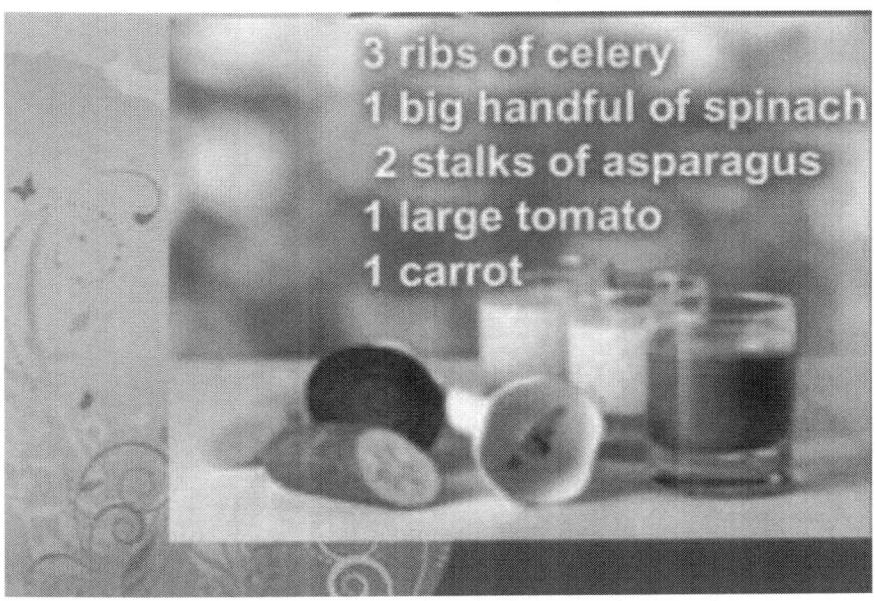

Are you looking for a full body cleanse and detox? I highly recommend this Green Tonic to wash out all the toxins from your system.

This Green Tonic is for you, if you love juices with some weird secret ingredient combinations that are super effective and that taste deliciously. You can always add a sweet apple if the taste is too strong for you.

Pouring the contents of a delightful juicy apple into your favorite blender and whip it all together into the most effective detox elixir is one of my favorite moments of the week.

This full body detoxer is very strong and I do not like to consume this juice every day. However, I make sure to at least consume this detoxing drink once per week.

If you are following an intensive full body cleanse program, this type of juice is what you want to aim for.

www.facebook.com/healthysmoothierecipes

This drink cleanses your system so that your body functions are going to work more productively after this strong elexir. It flushes out water, waste and toxins and helps boost up your system.

The full body detoxer contains the following ingredients:

Ingredients:

3 ribs of celery (organic if possible)

1 big handful of spinach (organic if possible or organic baby spinach)

2 stalks of asparagus (organic if possible)

1 large tomato (organic if possible)

1 carrot (organic if possible)

Directions:

For all these juice recipe For the directions please refer to the chapter where I am talking about my 5 Minute 6 Step Juicing System.

Here is a short instruction that sums up what to do. Make sure to refer back to my 6 step process for juicing so that you get the whole idea of juicing.

In this case peel the tomato, carrot and the asparagus.

Next cut and chop the veggies.

Put all the fruits and veggies from the ingredients list into your favorite juicer or blender or a combination of juicer/blender (Nutribullet) and strictly follow the directions of the manual that comes with your machine.

www.facebook.com/healthysmoothiesrecipes

Your blender manual will tell you what buttons to push and what speed to use.

Juice the softer textures first.

You will see that when you are juicing the crunchier veggies they will help you push the softer and more delicate ones through the blades.

Juice and blend all the ingredients from the list above together as per instructions.

Enjoy the Full Body Detoxer!

www.facebook.com/healthysmoothierecipes

Green Gold Juice

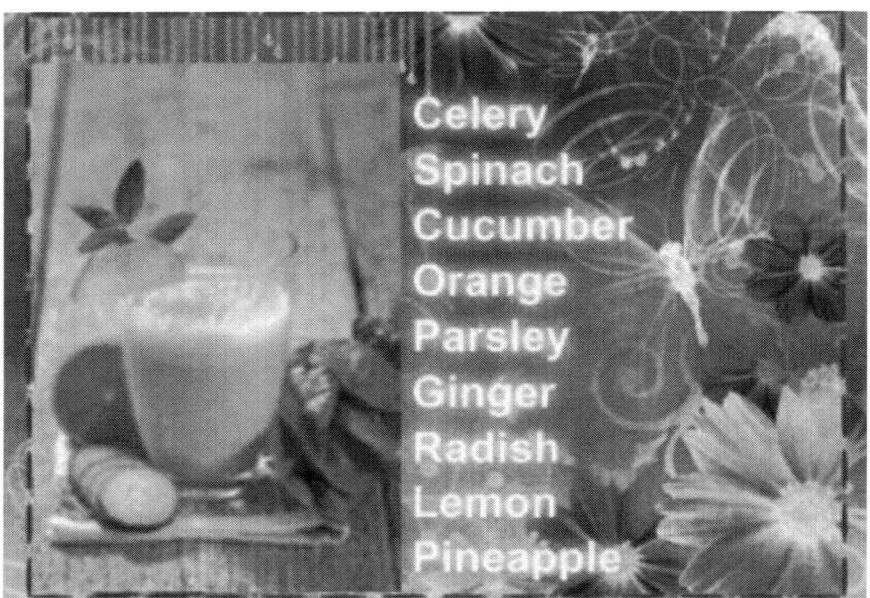

The ingredients of this powerful juice are all very beneficial for the body and brain.

Spinach is one of the most nutrient dense packed foods you can provide your body with. It proves you with energy. Spinach helps you fill your stomach without adding a lot of calories and you feel satisfied and full.

Spinach contains phytonutrients that are working as antioxidants battling against the free radical damage.

By consuming spinach you are helping to nourish your body on a cellular level.

Spinach is a great ingredients for weight loss juices.

Spinach is also an alkaline powerhouse. Baby spinach is great, too. Since there are so many other alkalizing vegetables out there, I recommend trying out different variations and concoct a juice that will send your pH levels to the sky.

This is also the reason why I love combining spinach and kale or baby spinach with spinach and kale.

The health benefits of celery are very powerful, too. In addition to being an alkaline food, celery is very low in calories and it is a great weight loss ingredient for juicing if weight loss is on your mind.

Celery is a great combination as a third ingredient because it brings even more health benefits to the table.

I always love to add celery into fruit based juices as well because it adds a bit of spiciness without overshadowing the sweet flavors of the fruits.

Experimenting with and knowing the benefits of all these ingredients is key to a successful juicing experience.

Parsley is the third green raw ingredient that powers up this juice drink to the next level. Parsley also helps keep your body alkaline. This green herb is not only powering up your juice with lots of health nutrients, but it helps bring out the freshest taste ever. It freshs up the taste of your juice because it adds more vitamins and minerals to your juice.

The great thing is that you can grow your own parsley pretty easily at home and always have it ready to freshen up your juices, smoothies and other recipes that you are making.

I only grow my own parsley and include it in most of my juicing drinks.

The fourth green ingredient of this power packed juice is the cucumber. The cucumber is a heavy hitter. I always keep a good stock of cucumbers at home. Cucumbers are alkaline, and they do contain so much water that it is a very hydrating vegetable.

The radish is very rich in folic acids and Vitamine C and even anthocyanins. These nutrients make the radish a very effective fighting food against cancer. Radish is effective in fighting oral cancer, intestinal cancer and colon cancer as well as stomach and kidney cancers.

Radishes also do contain Zinc, Vitamin C, and B-complex vitamins and phosphorus which is effective in treating skin disorders such as dry skin and rashes.

Radish juices are good for your digestive system and soothes it. Radish is a powerful detoxer and cleans your entire body from toxins. It helps to relieve the congestion of the respiratory system, too.

Radish juice is an excellent ingredients for asthmatic individual. People who are suffering from sinus and/or bronchial infections should tap into the healing power of radish.

It is beneficial for both the liver functions and the gallbladder because it acts as a cleaning agent.

Radish also contains sulphur based chemicals. This helps regulate the production and the flow of bile and bilirubin, acids and enzymes.

It also helps get rid of the excess bilirubin contained in the blood. Radish acts as a powerful detoxifying agent for your entire body.

Lastly, radish is highly effective in treating jaundice. Radish is able to halt the destruction of the red blood cells while increasing the supply of the blood's oxygen.

I highly recommend to use black radish for treating jaundice because it is stronger.

Radish is also a natural diuretic. It is very effective in fighting and preventing urinary tract infections. Radish juices do help to cure the burning feeling of the urinary tract. It helps heal bladder infections because it is the perfect natural kidney cleanser.

As you can see this juicing drink is a loaded with powerful ingredients that you can mix up and find lots of variations that might work for you.

I like adding some zesty ginger, orange and lemon to this power cocktail which makes the bitter taste of the celery and radish sweeter and like this you can transform it into the perfect healthy morning and breakfast booster.

The Green Gold Juice contains the following ingredients:

Ingredients:

4 Stalks of celery (organic if possible)

1 Cup of Spinach or baby spinach (organic if possible)

2 Cucumber (organic if possible)

1 Orange (organic if possible)

A few sprigs of parsley (organic if possible)

1 small knob of ginger (organic if possible)

1 small radish (organic if possible)

1 lemon (organic if possible)

1 big slice of pineapple

Directions:

www.facebook.com/healthysmoothierecipes

For all these juice recipe For the directions please refer to the chapter where I am talking about my 5 Minute 6 Step Juicing System.

Here is a short instruction that sums up what to do. Make sure to refer back to my 6 step process for juicing so that you get the whole idea of juicing.

In this case peel the radish, pineapple, ginger, orange, lemon, and cucumber.

Next cut and chop the fruits and veggies.

Put all the fruits and veggies from the ingredients list into your favorite juicer or blender or a combination of juicer/blender (Nutribullet) and strictly follow the directions of the manual that comes with your machine.

The manual will tell you what buttons to push and what speed to use.

Juice the softer textures first.

You will see that when you are juicing the crunchier veggies and fruits they will help you push the softer and more delicate fruits and veggies through the blades.

If you are not using a juicer and only have a blender available, make sure to first strain the juice from the lemon and orange.

Once it is finished you can either leave the pulp inside or take it out. This is totally up to your preference.

In this case you have to add the juice back to the blender and proceed from there.

Juice and blend the juices with the other ingredients from the list above together as per instructions.

www.facebook.com/healthysmoothiesrecipes

You can always add some raw honey or sweetener depending on your goal with these juices. If the juice is too strong for you, you might also add some ice cubes or source water.

Enjoy your Green Gold Juice!

Beet & Black Radish Liver Cleanser

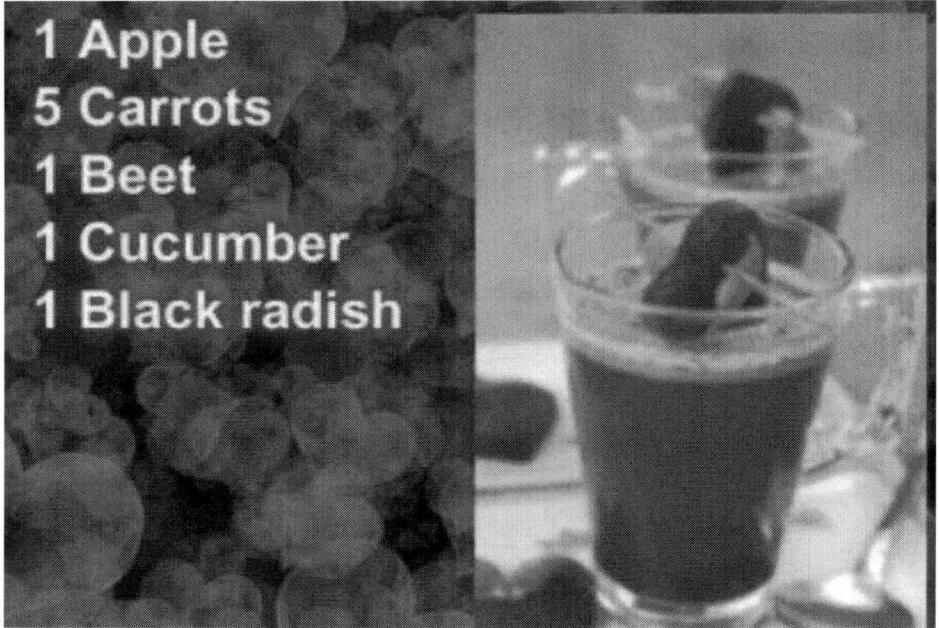

This beetroot liver cleanser contains a combination of healthy and cleansing cucumbers, beets, black radish and carrots. The secret of this juice comes from the combination.

The beets, carrots and cucumber are all nutrient-rich and packed with antioxidants and this is what makes this juice so powerful. This drink is a true immune system booster. It also is a powerful liver cleanse and detox drink because it cleans your system and makes it toxin free.

Beets provide the body with a rich source of Vitamin C and a wide range of other health benefits. The beetroot also contains folate and this helps prevent cancer and heart diseases.

The carrots enhance your vision health. Carrots provide you with a rich supply of antioxidant nutrients called beta carotene.

Cucumbers contain so much water that it is a very hydrating vegetable which combines very well with the healing benefits of the beet and the carrots.

Lastly, radish is highly effective in treating jaundice. Radish is able to halt the destruction of the red blood cells while increasing the supply of the blood's oxygen.

This hydrating liver cleanser juice is the perfect power booster for hot summer days, in the morning and whenever your body needs a good supply of hydration and the Beet & Black Radish Liver Cleanser contains the following ingredients:

Ingredients:

1 Apple (organic if possible)

5 carrots (organic if possible)

1 beet (organic if possible)

1 cucumber (organic if possible)

1 black radish (organic if possible)

Directions:

For the directions please refer to the chapter where I am talking about my 5 Minute 6 Step Juicing System.
Here is a short instruction that sums up what to do. Make sure to refer back to my 6 step process for juicing so that you get the whole idea of juicing.

In this case peel the apple, the radish, the beets (or buy them already prepared and ready to use), carrots and cucumber.

Next cut and chop the veggies.

Put all the veggies from the ingredients list into your favorite juicer or blender or a combination of juicer/blender (Nutribullet) and strictly follow the directions of the manual that comes with your machine.

The manual will tell you what buttons to push and what speed to use.

Juice the softer textures first. You will see that when you are juicing the crunchier fruits and veggies first they will help you push the softer and more delicate ones through the blades.

Juice and blend all the ingredients from the list above together as per instructions.

Enjoy this refreshing and hydrating Beet and Black Radish Liver Cleanser!

www.facebook.com/healthysmoothiesrecipes

Exotic Strawberry Rasperry Vitality Drink

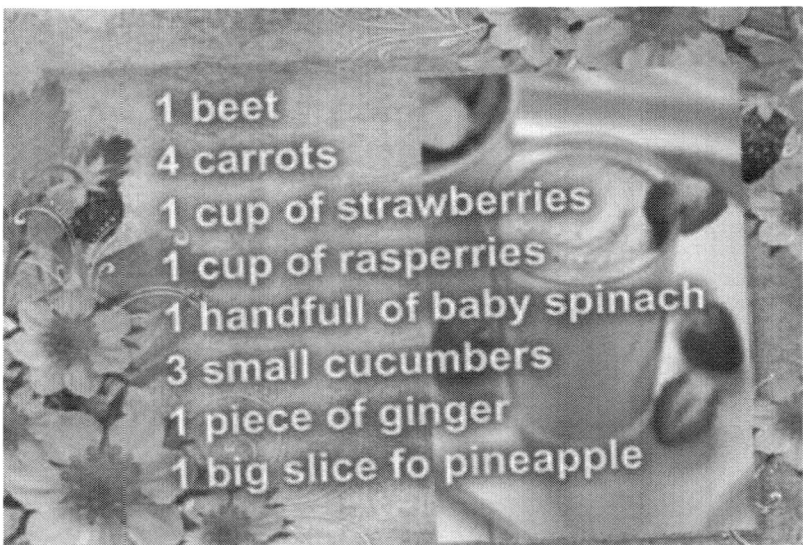

1 beet
4 carrots
1 cup of strawberries
1 cup of rasperries
1 handfull of baby spinach
3 small cucumbers
1 piece of ginger
1 big slice fo pineapple

Let's talk about a powerful combination of some fortified and nutritious red/orange superfoods like carrots, beets, strawberries and green superfoods.

The secret of this juice is the combination of the red/orange superfoods together with the greens.

This is a magical mixture of orange and green nutritious and healing vegetables and fruits. These are ingredients that do not only taste deliciously, but they will also give your body and brain the most powerful health benefits.

Carrots have a rich supply of antioxidant nutrients called beta carotene.

These delicious orange vegetables are the source not only of beta carotene, but also of a wide variety of antioxidants plus other health supporting nutrients.

www.facebook.com/healthysmoothierecipes

Other benefits of carrots are antioxidant benefits, cardiovascular benefits and vision for your health.

The real benefit of strawberries is that they are tasting great and that they are providing enough nutrients to the body.

Strawberries provide a boost to your immune system. They helps your eyes and they help fight cancer. They also helps with cholesterol and with inflammation. They also have anti-aging properties.

The mix of greens combined with orange and red raw fruits and veggies is what makes this juice so special.

The Exotic Strawberry Raspberry Vitality & Energy Booster contains the following ingredients:

Ingredients:

1 beet (organic if possible)

4 carrots (organic if possible)

1 cup of strawberries (organic if possible)

1 cup of raspberries (organic if possible)

1 handfull of baby spinach (organic if possible)

3 small cucumbers (organic if possible)

1 piece of ginger

1 big slice fo pineapple

Directions:

For all these juice recipe For the directions please refer to the chapter where I am talking about my 5 Minute 6 Step Juicing System.

Here is a short instruction that sums up what to do. Make sure to refer back to my 6 step process for juicing so that you get the whole idea of juicing.

In this case peel the ginger, beet (or buy already prepared and ready to use), carrots, pineapple, and cucumbers.

Next cut and chop the fruits and veggies.

Put all the fruits and veggies from the ingredients list into your favorite juicer or blender or a combination of juicer/blender (Nutribullet) and strictly follow the directions of the manual that comes with your machine.

The manual that comes with your machine will tell you what buttons to push and what speed to use.

Juice the softer textures first.

You will see that when you are juicing the crunchier veggies and fruits they will help you push the softer and more delicate fruits and veggies through the blades.

Juice and blend all the ingredients from the list above together as per instructions.

You can always add some raw honey or sweetener depending on your goal with these juices. If the juice is too strong for you, you might also add some ice cubes or source water.

Enjoy the delicious Exotic Strawberry Raspberry Vitality Drink!

www.facebook.com/healthysmoothierecipes

Notes

Natural Purple Energy Miracle

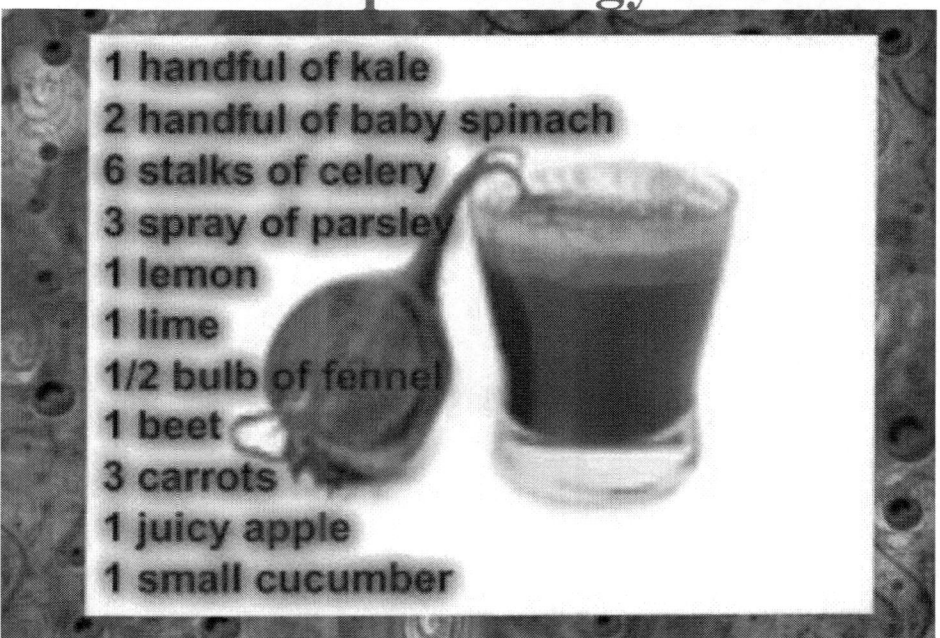

1 handful of kale
2 handful of baby spinach
6 stalks of celery
3 spray of parsley
1 lemon
1 lime
1/2 bulb of fennel
1 beet
3 carrots
1 juicy apple
1 small cucumber

The ingredients of the Natural Purple Energy Miracle Juice are all very beneficial for the body and brain.

The secret combination lies in the mix of red and green raw food ingredients.

The beetroot is one of the most healthy vegetables on earth. Consuming beets will help you feel energized. Beets are great for nourishing your brain. It can assist in lowering blood pressure.

Beets contain a very broad amount of minerals and vitamins. Add some beets to your juices to instantly up and power pack your nutrients without adding more calories or fat. It contains folate and this helps prevent cancer and heart diseases and Magnesium is keeping your energy levels up. It is also a very rich source of Vitamin C.

www.facebook.com/healthysmoothierecipes

The alkaline Kale combined with the beets makes an unbeatable juice cocktail that helps you reenergize and rejuvenate at the same time. I enjoy one of these whenever my energy levels are down.

The Natural Purple Energy Miracle contains the following ingredients:

Ingredients:

1 handful of kale (organic if possible)

2 handful spinach (organic if possible)

6 stalks of celery (organic if possible)

3 spray of parsley (organic if possible)

1 lemon (organic if possible)

1 lime (organic if possible)

½ bulb of fennel (organic if possible)

1 beet (organic if possible)

3 carrots (organic if possible)

Directions:

For all these juice recipe For the directions please refer to the chapter where I am talking about my 5 Minute 6 Step Juicing System.

Here is a short instruction that sums up what to do. Make sure to refer back to my 6 step process for juicing so that you get the whole idea of juicing.

www.facebook.com/healthysmoothiesrecipes

In this case peel the lemons, limes, carrots, and beet (or buy prepared).

Next cut and chop the fruits and veggies.

Put all the fruits and veggies from the ingredients list into your favorite juicer or blender or a combination of juicer/blender (Nutribullet) and strictly follow the directions of the manual that comes with your machine.

The manual will tell you what buttons to punch and what speed to use.

Juice the softer fruits/textures first.

You will see that when you are juicing the crunchier veggies and fruits they will help you push the softer and more delicate fruits and veggies through the blades.

If you are not using a juicer and only have a blender available, make sure to first strain the juice from the lemon and lime.

Once it is finished you can either leave the pulp inside or take it out. This is totally up to your preference.

In this case you have to add the juice back to the blender and proceed from there.

Juice and Blend the juices with the other ingredients from the list above together as per instructions.

You can always add some raw honey or sweetener depending on your goal with these juices. If the juice is too strong for you, you might also add some ice cubes or source water.

Enjoy your Red Kale Juice!

www.facebook.com/healthysmoothierecipes

Juicing For Vitality & Energy The Smart Way

These are some pro tips you can apply to these healthy smoothies to make your juicing habits even more effective:

1. Balance fruits and veggies because they are easier to eat on the run. In general, people eat more fruits than vegetables. When you are juicing, make sure to strive for a ratio of at least three parts of veggies and one part of fruits. This will help you to take in veggies while keeping your total sugar content under control.

2. Sweeten up your drink. Hearty greens like kale, beets, parsley and swiss chard, are bitter in taste and it helps to add some fruits like apples to sweeten up your juice. You can also try a spice like cinnamon or allspice.

If that is still not enough, drizzle a few drops of honey or maple syrup into your juice.

3. Drink your juice promptly. It is best to enjoy it immediately after the juicing process otherwise you will lose nutrients. Damage and loss or nutrients starts as soon as the drink is exposed to oxygen.

Just think about how quickly a slice of avocado or apple starts to get brown! It is therefore best to consume your juice no longer than 15 minutes after the juice is in your glass.

If you are preparing the juice for later make sure to store it for a short period of time in a mason jar with a very tight seal.

4. Never gulp down your juice, but drink it with the philosophy of mindfulness.

www.facebook.com/healthysmoothiesrecipes

Chewing" and Swishing the liquid before swallowing helps you with the digestion process. It also maximizes both satiety and assimilation.

5. Make sure to maintain quality control because you only want to stick to organic fruits and vegetables. You have to be aware that juicing does require a bigger amount of veggies and fruits than if you were just eating the same amount

Only use the most nutritious veggie and fruit varieties that you can find and concentrate on vegetables and fruits that are higher in beta-carotene and minerals than others. Always include veggies like cabbage, kale, romaine, and celery.

6. Never waste the plant parts of the veggies. The bases of broccoli and cauliflower and asparagus can be used for juicing. The stems and the leaves of beets are perfect for juicing, too.

7. The right tools can save you lots of time. Always make sure to look for a juicer that has a wide mouth. A mouth that is able to eject the pulp and that is easier to clean.

Having a fast juicer can make the difference between you enjoying juicing every day and you not enjoying juicing at all and quitting the whole idea of juicing.

This is why buying a quality juicer is critical for your whole juicing success.

8. As for blenders, keep in mind that blenders are not juicers. It is good to have a juicer and a blender, but keep in mind that blenders simply cannot make juices.

In addition to your daily juicing habits, keep eating whole natural foods, too, because juices alone are not enough.

You want to take in whole natural and organic foods

9. I encourage you to drink your Secret Morning Elixir, then your first morning juice and/or smoothie (depending on your goal) and eat whole foods on a daily basis.

Like this you make sure that you provide your body with a great nutrition, a high amount of fibers that comes from the whole foods as well as a complementary intake of micronutrients.

Effortless Juicing Process (Juicing Has Never Been Easier)

Preserve yourself from overeating by drinking a big cup of juices well before eating.

If you are able to pinpoint a juice extractor that is certainly high quality and operates on lower speeds, this would be your best choice. Increased speed might overheat your machine and thus destroy the nutrients of your juices.

Make sure to refer to the Green Star Juicer Review which has advantages as opposed to other juicers in relation to this overheating issue.

If you are in an age bracket over 50, you should be thinking to include juicing into your lifestyle in order to reduce the process of aging.

Pick a product or service which can be premium quality, simple to use and valued to match within your spending budget.

Add ginger to your juices and meal plan. Adding ginger to your juices also provides you with zesty flavor. Ginger also has a anti inflammatory quality. It helps you recover injuries.

Purchase a masticating juice extractor which will keep the nutrition in the juices that you are making.

If you prefer juices without the pulp, I recommend to use an espresso filtration system or some cheesecloth to filter out the pulp.

Make sure to always include green super foods like kale, broccoli and spinach into your juices and shoot for 50%-75% plant based ingredients plus some other veggies and fruits for

www.facebook.com/healthysmoothierecipes

the sweet flavoring and to balance the sometimes bitter flavor of the veggies.

Should you be juicing as a result of health problems, make sure to get started with dark green fruits and leafy vegetables as your basic juices.

Never use industrial fruit juices to replace real fruits because they are full of natural sweets and consist of much less nutrients and vitamins than fresh juices.

If you do not like the bitter taste of some veggies make sure to balance the flavor with fruits like apples. In my opinion apples like Fuji, Rome, and Gala are the providing the best flavour.

When attempting to lose weight with juicing, try to create pineapple liquid with your juicer and you will find that adding apples are a wonderful combination with pineapple juice.

If you are on a juicing diet, you may want to lower the calories by adding an equal amount of ice cubes or source water.

Make time for yourself to truly enjoy your juices and try to get a feel for the different ingredients and flavors.

Juicing is even much easier and much more fun when the entire family takes part in the process. Have a child wash the fruits and veggies while a grown-up chops and processes it. If you include your kids, you will keep them interested and integrated into a healthy lifestyle at an early age which will benefit the health of your child enormously. Imagine not having to run to the doctor for every disease the child might come up with!

Make sure to respect the amounts and the combination with real healthy food because juicing alone is not a solution. It is always meant in a way to substitute your healthy daily diet in order to keep you and your family fit based on the highly nutritious value that you will be supplied with from these healthy juices.

Make sure to research and know the benefits of the veggies and fruits that you are using. Every single vegetable and fruit gives distinct vitamins and nutrients and you must be aware what they do for you.

Improve your every day intake of nutrients by making juicing part of your eating habits. Your whole body will reap the benefits plus you will find that these juices are not only healthy and fat burning in nature, but these juices are also super easy to make and taste deliciously.

Juicing is a simple to acquire skill and if you turn this skill into a habit, you will be able to live a clean, toxin free and lean life from the inside out and for a very long time.

Juicing keeps the doctor away and doubles your life!

www.facebook.com/healthysmoothierecipes

Power Up Your Juicing Habits With Healing & Detoxifiying Wheat Grass Elixirs

Wheat grass is simply put a young wheat plant. Wheat grass is widely consumed in liquid form by health conscious people who prefer the concentrated rich source of enzymes, minerals and vitamins.

The main aspect that makes these wheat grass juices so healthy is the fact that it contains chlorophyll.

Nearly 70% of wheat grass is chlorophyll. Some individual state that a small pound of wheat grass is equal to 20 pounds of fresh garden greens! This is just one of the reason why health fans are liquefying this grass and drinking it.

Wheat grass juice is quickly rising to the top of the favorite juices.

It retains most of the essential minerals. These minearls, enzymes and vitamins are promoting health and help repair cell damage.

Wheat grass juice also has the ability to increase oxygenation in the human body plus it helps build up the red blood cells. These red blood cells are the carriers of oxygen to the body's cells. In addition it purifies our blood and organs while destroying the nasty toxins. In general, wheat grass is a true metabolism booster.

Wheat grass juice is the perfect replacement for dark green leafy vegetables that you should supplement your diet with.

www.facebook.com/healthysmoothiesrecipes

Wheatgrass is also a very rich source of alkalinity for the body. It is often found in supplemental form so that you can mix it with water and drink it if you do not have an adequate juicer that can process wheat grass.

Some fans choose to drink a daily glass of fresh wheatgrass juice to insure that their body is getting enough alkaline forming food.

Juicers can break down the cellulose barriers and extract all of the juice inside fruits, grasses and veggies.

However, you should know that not all juicers are capable of making real wheat grass juice.

If you try to juice wheat grass in a juicer that is not made to process grass, you will probably end up with a damaged or clogged juicer.

The best juicers for wheat grass are those that are multipurpose juicers. These multipurpose juicers will not only make juices from veggies and fruits, but you can apply them to make wheat grass.

If you have any questions, simply ask lots of questions before buying your juicer.

You may want to purchase a wheat grass juicer if you plan to only process grass. These juicers are also known as single auger juicers. They are crushing the grass while squeezing out all of the rich chlorophyll juice of the grass.

Newer models of these single auger juicers do include two levels. The first level works to crush the grass and squeeze out the healthy juice while the second level pulls the remaining pulp through a second crushing and extraction process.

Today you can find many models of these auger or juice extractors. Do not let buying a juicer get in your way. Simply identify what type of juicer you want by determining what type of ingredients you want to process.

Remember, when you get into the habit of drinking healthy wheat grass juice, you should go step by step and start out slowly because the taste of the wheat juice migh surprise you at first.

I did not like the taste at all when I got started, but learned how to integrate these healthy green juices into my daily juicing ritual.

I started by drinking one ounce per day and slowly work my way up to three ounces per day which is the perfect amount in order to get the most nutritious value into the system of the body.

You will see that such a habit will bring long term health and a clean and lean body!

Green Star Juicer Review

Staying healthy is something that is directly related to having good eating habits, an effective organization of your daily chores and a balanced lifestyle.

In my opinion it also entails a balanced food choice and diet plan that is rich in all types of nutrients. The right amount of nutrients is also important.

Juicers like the Green Star juicer have become extremely popular and important in modern society so that people can be able to balance their food choices in a healthier and more effective way.

However, the market for any kind of juicers these days is too large in order to make a smart choice from the get go and without being informed. Before you actually purchase any juicer, you should actually go through the benefits and features of the juicer that you consider.

In my view the Green Star Juicer is a good choice even though I prefer the Breville.

It is my duty to inform you about a second option that is available to you and that you might consider as a second choice if you do not want to go with the Breville.

The following is a list of items to expect with the purchase of a Green Star juicer.

Retractable Plug Green Star Juicer:

It is very likely that when you operate the machine without reading the instructions, you will not be able to find the plug.

This is a very common error because the plug and the wire extension of these Green Star Juicers do have their own designated place inside the juicer itself because the juicer has a retractable plug.

Solid Body Green Star Juicer:

The first thing you notice when you see or touch a Green Star juicer is that it is made to be of durable and stable materials.

It is based on a very balanced construction and everything is efficiently located and equated with this juicer.

Since juicers and similar products tend to be on the expensive side of things, it is very important that you take a look on the quality of the materials and the durability.

Heat Transfer Green Star Juicer:

The heat transfer from the machine to the juicer is a major issue with most juicers because heat transfer can destroy the nutrients in the veggies and fruits.

This juicer has a slow two-gear system. This system is critical and crucial to the quality of the juice.

You should really take a closer look before making your final decision because this juicer has some critical, indiscutable and obvious benefits.

Array of Attachments Green Star Juicer:

There are very important applications for the Green Star juicer in pasta making as well. If you are a pasta lover this is absolutely for you!

This is why taking a closer look at the Green Star Juicer if you are looking to buy a food processor at the same time.

www.facebook.com/healthysmoothiesrecipes

This juicer is available in a wide array of attachments. This fact alone will increase the application of this juicer which in turn makes this option a very good solution in terms of the value that you are getting for your money.

Warranty Green Star Juicer:

Another big advantage of the Green Star juicer is that it comes with a five years attached warranties.

This means that if there is some kind of problem in this period then you can get it fixed without any problems.

Final Verdict For The Green Star Juicer:

A Green Star juicer is an extremely loaded machine that will not only improve the quality of life with regards to taste and quality of nutrition, but it also gives you a huge array of variety like making pasta and processing other types of food.

The 5 year warranty is yet another benefit that is almost unmatched by the industry and this is a real competitive advantage over the other products that only offer 1 year warranties.

Breville Speed Juice Extractor Review

Juicing is one of the most popular health trends at the moment. It detoxifies the body system. Juicing gives you a strong dose of nutrients and vitamins and minerals.

Juicing can even help you lose weight and maintain a healthy living. If you are interested in a juicing diet, I recommend a juice extractor. A juice extractor will be a helpful, usable and valuable addition to your daily food plan and lifestyle.

There is a big choice of juicers available and it can be a difficult process to determine which juicer is best for you. After looking at the numerous accessories, advantages, features and user reviews.

In my view it is clear as day that the Breville BJE510XL Ikon Juicer is the best choice because it has consistently performed better and more effective than the competing juicers. The Breville is one of the best juice extractors on the market today.

Juicing Performance Of The Breville

You want to make sure that your juicer is able to extract juice from fruits and veggies without leaving much of excess pulp behind. The Breville BJE510XL will perform in this respect. It extracts only the optimal amount of nutritious juice from veggies and fruits.

Ikon Jucier Overview of The Breville:

900 watts
Measures 16 x 9 x 16 inches
5-speed system
Speeds range from 6500 rpm to 12500 rpm
Weighs 9 pounds

Volume Level Of The Breville:

The Breville seems to generate the same amount of noise as the competitors like the Green Star Juicer and others.

The noise will depend on your individual noise tolerance. You can expect it to make the same level of noise as an average juicer or blender.

Speed Of The Breville:

The Breville BJE510XL is designed with a speed control. The speed of the machine can be adapted to the veggies and fruits that are used. When you are juicing with the Breville, veggies and soft fruits do require a slower speed than firmer and crunchier fruits and veggies like broccoli. The Breville is designed with a control that allows you to effectively run the machine at exactly the right speed to get the most out of the juice.

www.facebook.com/healthysmoothierecipes

It is designed to use the minimum effort to achieve the maximum results. The Breville also comes with a user friendly manual. The manual tells you the exact speed that you should set for each ingredient. This gives you the maximum output of juice and a minimum of messing around.

Juicer Design Of The Breville:

The Breville has a large shoot. It is spacious enough to fit several carrots or a whole apple in at a time. This reduces the time you can spend and it takes away the tedious tasks of slicing, dicing and chopping.

This juicer is something you are going to be proud to show off in your home. It has a very sleek and stainless steel finishing which will complement almost any home decor. The classy design earned a designer prize, the Australian Design Award.

Another feature of the Breville which contributes to the look is the fact that it will not stain after usage. Many juicers become discolored after usage, but the Breville BJE510XL is easy to clean and always returns into its original appearance after usage.

The Breville Juicer comes with several parts. It creates a firm seal when all the parts are snapped together. The juicer comes with a bright LCD screen. The LCD screen shows your current settings with fruit icons. This will guide you to select the matching speed for each ingredient.

www.facebook.com/healthysmoothiesrecipes

What Comes With The Breville?

When you buy the Breville juicer you get a manual, a juice jug, a detachable spout, a froth separator and a cleaning brush.

Clean Up Of The Breville

Many consumers do love the Breville juicer because it is especially easy to clean up. When it is running, you will notice that all of the pulp is deposited into a separate container. If this separate container is lined with plastic, it will quickly and easily be able to be emptied out. The various parts of the Breville juicer easily disassemble and fit easily into your dishwasher.

Warranty Of The Breville?

1 year of replacement warranty comes with the Breville BJE510XL juicer.

www.facebook.com/healthysmoothierecipes

Juicing For Vitality Quiz

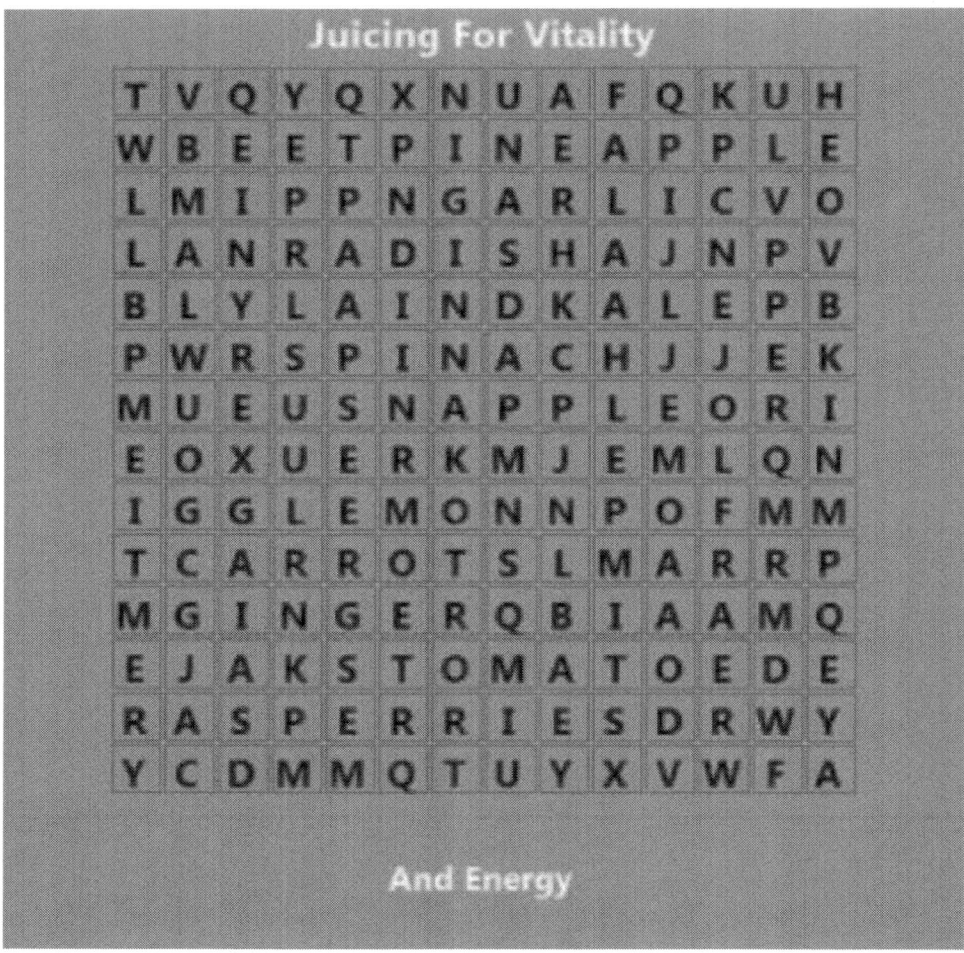

All you have to do is find 12 juicing ingredient related words. Use your imagination, read backwards, sidewards, and forwards to find the correct Juicing related words and associations. Go to the next page to see the correct answers!

Have fun:)

www.facebook.com/healthysmoothiesrecipes

www.facebook.com/healthysmoothierecipes

Answers

Quiz Answers:

1. **Orange**
2. **Apple**
3. **Lime**
4. **Ginger**
5. **Kale**
6. **Celery**
7. **Carrots**
8. **Beets**
9. **Strawberries**
10. **Spinach**
11. **Parsley**
12. **Fennel**

www.facebook.com/healthysmoothiesrecipes

Conclusion

I have a lot of fun experimenting with these juicing recipes and I hope that these same recipes are getting you started with your own vitality and energy juicing goals, too.

There's a lot of satisfaction when you stumble on a healthy juicing recipe that tastes fantastic, too. It's even more gratifying if the recipe is 5 minute quick and simple to make at the same time.

Don't be afraid to add or remove ingredients to make the recipe your own and as Ann Wigmore, one of the front-runners of today's raw food movement, declared, "Be creative; you just need to understand approximately what to do."

When you do make changes, jot them down! There is little worse than playing around and making a great recipe only to realize you can't remember precisely what you probably did. By making juices that you adore, you'll find yourself anticipating your juice breakfast or juice break.

Since they're so high in nourishment, you will begin to feel more fit.

If you're like me, you may also find that the more that you drink juices, the more that you will begin to enjoy healthier food options like salads and fresh items. Convenience foods like potato chips will begin to taste tasteless.

The additional energy you get from the fruit, vegetable and plant based juices will also assist you in working out more.

All this will assist you in making your juicing efforts a big success!

www.facebook.com/healthysmoothierecipes

I attempted to make this Juicing For Vitality & Energy system as easy, fascinating, inspiring, easy to use and as practical to

consume as possible for you because a system like this has to be compatible with today's fast paced and mobile world.

Just keep the book on your portable gadget next to your working table and go through one recipe at a time and as you progress with your own juicing goals for health, vitality and energy.

Make it a fun and exciting challenge and stick to it. Remember changing your eating and drinking habits is becoming easier and easier as time goes by and as you get used to your new juicing habits. This is a marathon and not a sprint. It is important to take your time in order to change your habits, improve, and adapt to this new juicing lifestyle!

The book is intended to be used in an interactive and stimulating fashion and to empower you to take action at the same time.

Remember the juices are 5 minute quick to prepare so this even works for the busiest person in the world.

Ultimately, the goal of this book is to lead you to a healthy lifestyle that includes healthy and nutritious juices and food choices.

Including these healthy juicing drinks into your daily meal plans and including them into your lifestyle is what you should be aiming for as your ultimate goal.

Once you are at the level of including healthy juices into your daily lifestyle, you have achieved a big success towards a healthy lifestyle because your body uses the natural healing power of these plant based foods and superfoods that are contained in these juices.

www.facebook.com/healthysmoothiesrecipes

Your body will be able to provide protection and fight infections and viruses. It will be able to heal itself, boost your vitality and energy and ultimately safe you from lots of pain, diseases and expensive doctor bills.

This is a goal that you will never be able to achieve with some common food alternatives or fancy meal plans. Following the latest food trends that are popular is a plan for error and disaster and you do not want to be a victim of these chemically, sick making, and industrially fabricated food design products..

The plan of this Juicing for vitality and energy lifestyle, however, is very kind and intelligent because it follows the rules and the creativity of the nature and the body. It nourishes and energizes the body throughout the day with all the beneficial ingredients and nutrients that are beneficial for the body and mind and it keeps your body and mind productive all the time.

I hope you will use and consume the content whenever you need some inspiration and motivation for making some healthy juice drinks that are helping you live the healthy lifestyle.

Remember, all you have to do is open the book and start with the first juice drink preparation.

Go through all of them and apply them on a daily basis as you see fit and depending on the health goal that you are looking to achieve.

Remember to get started every morning with the Secret Morning Elixir first before drinking your first juice in order to accelerate the health benefits that come with juicing.

You will soon see for yourself that making these juices is a lot of fun plus a lifestyle with juices is going to make you very happy, satisfied, balanced, fit, and energized!

www.facebook.com/healthysmoothierecipes

Double your vitality, energy, and life today by the power of juicing!

To your success,

Juliana Baldec

www.facebook.com/healthysmoothiesrecipes

More Information

If you enjoy my work, please feel free to join our facebook pages at:

http://www.facebook.com/howtomeditatevideos

http://www.facebook.com/pages/Yoga-For-Beginners/483214588418927

http://www.facebook.com/healthysmoothierecipes

Alecandra Baldec's Official Website:

http://www.howtomeditatevideos.com

You can also follow us on Twitter and Youtube at:

https://twitter.com/alecandrabaldec

http://www.youtube.com/user/howtomeditatevideos

And if you are interested in learning more about our other products and publications, please visit:

Alecandra Baldec's Yoga & Meditation Books:

Alecandra Baldec's Yoga & Meditation lifestyle books here

Juliana Baldec's Books:

Juliana Baldec's Yoga Books

To keep yourself updated and to claim your Bonus please visit my healthy smoothie recipe Facebook page here: http://www.facebook.com/healthysmoothiesrecipes

Best wishes in your endeavors!

Juliana Baldec

Notes

www.facebook.com/healthysmoothierecipes

More Information

If you enjoy my work, please feel free to join our facebook pages at:

http://www.facebook.com/howtomeditatevideos

http://www.facebook.com/pages/Yoga-For-Beginners/483214588418927

http://www.facebook.com/healthysmoothiesrecipes

Alecandra Baldec's Official Website:

[#http://www.howtomeditatevideos.com

You can also follow us on Twitter and Youtube at:

https://twitter.com/alecandrabaldec

http://www.youtube.com/user/howtomeditatevideos

www.facebook.com/healthysmoothiesrecipes

And if you are interested in learning more about our other products and publications, please visit:

Alecandra Baldec's Yoga & Meditation Books:

Just type into Amazon.com: Alecandra Baldec

Juliana Baldec's Books:

Just type into Amazon.com: Juliana Baldec

Best wishes in your endeavors!

Juliana Baldec

www.facebook.com/healthysmoothierecipes

Smoothies Are Like You

The Smoothie Lifestyle & Smoothie Diet In 25 Rhymes: From A to Z

Smoothies are a refreshing drink to have every day.
They help your body in many amazing ways!
You can restore or rejuvenate or even lose weight.
Yes, Smoothies are always something quite great!

How great can smoothie be?

Let's take a look from A to Z!

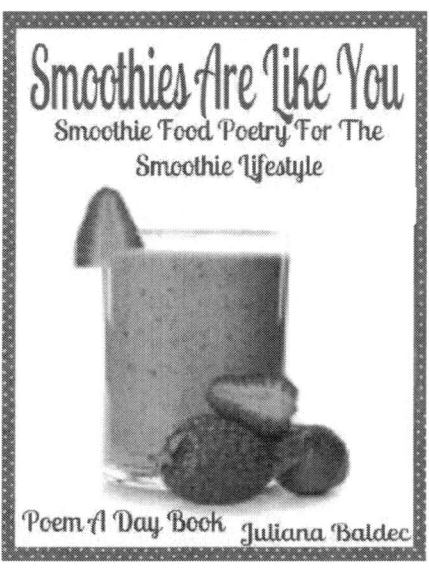

Are you ready to learn about the Smoothie Lifestyle from A to Z?
If so, then come along, let's learn about the raw Smoothie laws just you and me..

www.facebook.com/healthysmoothiesrecipes

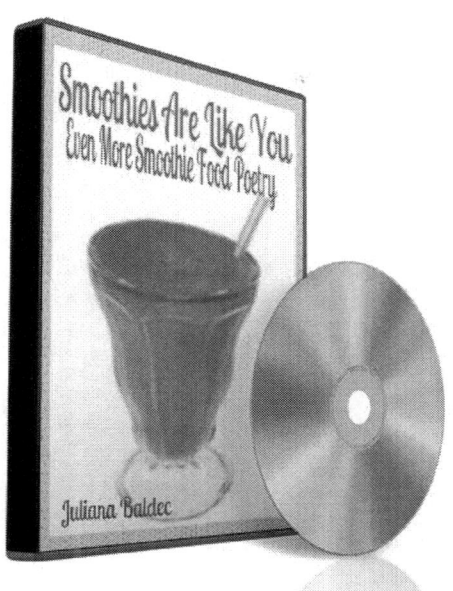

LIMITED-TIME SPECIAL: Special Bonus...

That's right...For a limited time you can download even More Smoothies Are Like You Moments...

To get access, please click the link below...

Unforgettable Smoothie Pleasures
http://ohmyfavoritethings.com

or

http://www.facebook.com/healthysmoothiesrecipes

Why Smoothie Poems?

Juliana Baldec's "Smoothies Is Like You" is an extremely fun, quick and easy to read little rhyming book about the amazing Smoothie Lifestyle. It is for everyone no matter if you are looking for information about the Smoothie diet for beginners or if you are an advanced Smoothie consumer.

This little food poetry Smoothie lifestyle book gives everyone who thinks the healthy Smoothie lifestyle is great some effective and straight forward universal Smoothie guidance and advice in a very funny and rhyming way.

This Smoothie food poem a day book is not only a fun way to discover the way of Smoothies, but it also gives some great inspirational and motivational insights into your health.

These Smoothie moments are divided into 25 poems and classified from A like Smoothies are like Albert Einstein to Smoothis are like Z and like Smoothie Zone.

Enjoying these rhyming Smoothie foody poems can teach many ways to embrace that enjoyable Smoothie way of life. It can also teach many ways to accept a healthier nutrition in general and to manage and overcome negative emotions like guilt & sacrifice and other emotionally painful moments that come with overeating and eating unhealthy rich food and that are relate to eating and enjoying food.

Reading these Smoothie lifestyle rhymes about the Smoothie Lifestyle & the Smoothie Diet that go from A to Z teaches many ways how to integrate the Smoothie lifestyle into your way of live to find a healthy balanced nutrition, happiness, fitness, and a lean and clean body.

www.facebook.com/healthysmoothiesrecipes

Juliana uses the simple form of rhymes to encourage even beginners of the Smoothie diet to discover their way of Smoothies in a fun, unorthodox and unconventional way.

Juliana shows that everyone and even the most busy person can read these easy to consume Smoothie food poems and get something valuable out of it. This interesting and intriguing food for thought touches everyone's life because Smoothies are about health and happiness and no matter what one knows already about the fascinating world of Smoothies, Smoothie lovers will guaranteed find some inspiration in this fun little book for the Smoothie soul.

The book encourages everyone who is interested in healthy, raw, vegan, lean and clean superfoods and eating and drinking to take a peek inside and be inspired by the many ways of the Smoothie lifestyle. This "Smoothie Is Like You" book can be used in an unlimited way to help you become healthier and happier - just like the many ways of the Smoothie lifestyle that you will discover inside!

The one who makes the most creative use of the book is the one who will find the most value in it because there is truly an unlimited amount of applications and uses for this helpful little poem a day book.

You could take one poem a day and reflect upon it. You could use a poem and gift it to a loved one who is a Smoothie lover to show your gratitude or just say thank you in a unique way. You could also use a specific poem to prove a point or to give encouragement, inspiration and motivation to someone you love and who is looking for more information about the Smoothie diet for beginners.

You could play with the letters. For example, if you like someone whose name is Adam, you could take the first poem called Smoothies are Like A and give it to that person to express your gratitude. You can do the same thing with all the letters and gift the poem to someone you like to surprise with a a personalized name Smoothie poem. Giving little gratitude and thank you gifts like that in order to show your attention, affection and love for someone you care about is a wonderful way to socialize and to share your own passions for the Smoothie lifestyle.

You could also use the poems as an inspiration to write your own inspirational Smoothie journal that incudes your own journey with Smoothies and all of your favorite Smoothie recipes.

Some creative crafters are even using them to make their own personal Smoothie scrapbooking recipe books, notebooks, calendars, photo journals, quote clipping books, and you name it.

You can do whatever your creative heart desires and as long as you are using the poems only for your own personal usage and joy you can do whatever you like.

Poems include Famous Smoothie quotes as well as quotes relating to health and happiness by Anthony Robbins, Darwin, Johnny Carson, Buddha, Mother Teresa, Oscar Wilde and many more. They are organized by names and from A to Z in coherence with the poems.

The collection of poems includes 25 Smoothie poems from A to Z with quotes just like this one:

"The higher your energy level, the more efficient your body. The more efficient your body, the better you feel and the more you will use your talent to produce outstanding results." -Anthony Robbins

The book encourages everyone to start their own journey of the Smoothie lifestyle and it concludes with some very encouraging thoughts so that everyone can choose to start and continue his or her own path of the Smoothie Lifestyle. The book helps with the discovery phase of Smoothies and opens the doors for more discovery.

The ultimate goal is to encourage people who read this Smoothie poem a day book to get started and to anticipate their own journey and their own Smoothie ritual. The start is always the and most difficult step. If you are open and willing to take that first step you will find the Smoothie Lifestyle your way.

Juliana helps with the discovery phase of Smoothies via the direction of inspirational and motivational poems and quotes so that everyone is enabled to live a healthy and happy lifestyle with Smoothies.

The book is designed to awaken your own inner voice, your own creativity and your own individuality to use the book for your own personal Smoothie expression.

The book has tons of applications and usability and it there for you to do what every your own goals with Smoothies might be.

Turning your discovery of the many ways of Smoothies that you are brought in touch with inside the book into your own way of using Smoothies is what this journey is all about. Juliana encourages you to discover all the aspects of Smoothies in an intriguing, appealing, fun and rhyming way and tries to connect you with your inner Smoothie self so that you will find your own direction and your own way of the Smoothie Lifestyle.

Sustaining yourself and growing into a healthy and happy lean and clean body and mind is only one aspect and benefit of the way of the Smoothie lifestyle that you will profit from once you accept the law of the Smoothie lifestyle into your own life. The book also brings you in touch and stimulates you with the many possibilities of Smoothies. Once you get in touch with the many ways of Smoothies, you will see that you will find an unlimited

www.facebook.com/healthysmoothierecipes

amount of the most amazing Smoothie moments, and this is where the real fun begins!

This will be the most unforgettable journey of your life so if you are curious and intrigued about the Smoothie lifestyle, or if you are already advanced, make sure to pick up this Paleo food poetry because you will guaranteed broaden your knowledge about many other fascinating ways of the Smoothie lifestyle.

You will for sure get in touch with some intriguing, fascinating and curious ways that you have not yet considered.

Smoothies are all about leading a healthy and happy lifestyle like our ancestors did, and even if you think you don't have time for Smoothie stuff like this because you are busy or because you just don't believe in it, you will be amazed how different this little inspirational and fun Smoothie poem a day book really can be. It will open your eyes and it will open your heart and it will open your mind to the most wonderous and fascinating thing in the world:

Your own health and happiness via the Smoothie lifestyle!

Make sure to take your health seriously because there is nobody else who will do it for you. You are your own master of creating your own health and happiness!

This book is all about yourself and finding your proper path of nutrition and clean eating and drinking and that is why this book is so fascinating because it is about yourself AKA "Smoothies Are Like You".

It is the perfect little poem for mom or poem for dad gift that you can give to anyone who you love and it is even a great gift idea for a child who can
already read because these funny rhyming verses of the Smoothie lifestyle are a great way to have fun and learn at the same time.

www.facebook.com/healthysmoothiesrecipes

The earlier you start your discovery phase of your own health and the many ways of Smoothies the better the quality of your body and life is going to become in the future. If you love your child, discover the many ways of Smoothies via one poem a day with him or her because you can not give them a more valuable gift than making them aware of the unlimited possibilities that life with a healthy lifestyle like Smoothies or any other healthy nutrition can bring them.

Make sure to get this fun and inspirational Smoothie poem a day and Smoothie quote book today because nothing is more important than your own health and that of your loved ones!

Dedication

For my parents who are the most important health influencers in my life!

You have my unconditional love, always!

www.facebook.com/healthysmoothierecipes

Smoothies Are Like A

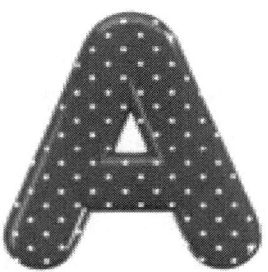

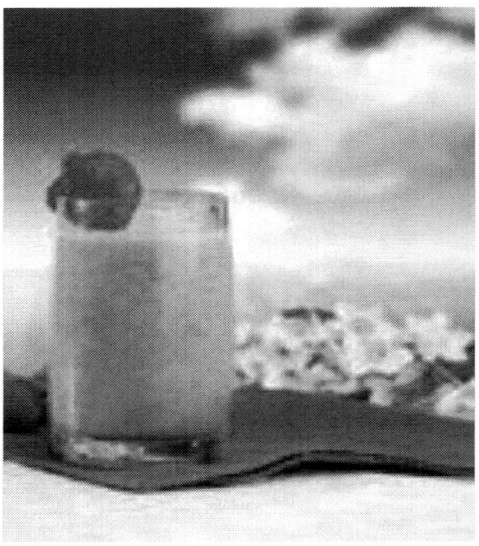

Smoothies remind me a lot of the letter A because Smoothies are like Albert Einstein, just slightly insane.
They are of course healthier to drink than Champagne because Smoothies are good for your brain.
Just make sure you never get your Smoothie from the discount chain or with sugar cane because you want yours with kale or romaine.

www.facebook.com/healthysmoothiesrecipes

These green ones are really good for you because they maintain your superior thyroid vein.

The ones without grain are the best to gain health and are good for your cell membrane.

Remember, you can always find recipes in the public domain.

The undisputed and hard hitting truth with Smoothies is just like this.

Smoothies are not only good for your brain they are also keeping you sane.

If you don't believe me here is what Anthony Robbins has to say to this:

"The higher your energy level, the more efficient your body. The more efficient your body, the better you feel and the more you will use your talent to produce outstanding results." -Anthony Robbins

Paleo makes outstanding results with your body possible!

www.facebook.com/healthysmoothierecipes

Smoothies Are Like B

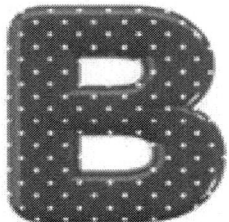

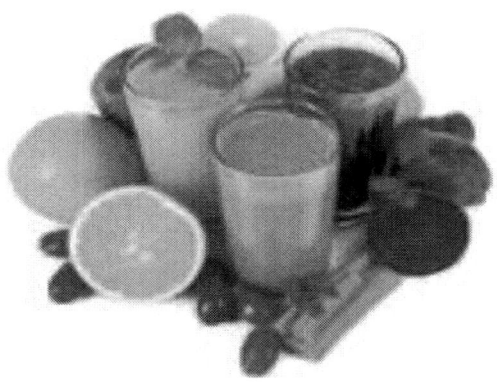

Smoothies are pretty much like the letter B because Smoothies have great benefits, like supercharged nutrient goodness.
You can use fruits and vegetables because not only are they more credible, but vegetables are also tasty and edible.
Smoothies are spectacularly incredible because they are vegetal and far from chemical.
If you'll ask a health professional they will tell you Smoothies are indefensible and indispensable.
Health professionals will also tell you that these unforgettable delectable drinks are a helpfully heavenly remedy.
Don't you agree?

www.facebook.com/healthysmoothiesrecipes

Smoothies are just an unforgettable and delectable spectacle!

Let me tell you this. If you stick to it, you will never get sick!

Budda can really speak to this because he has the experience:

"Every human being is the author of his or her own health or disease." -Bhudda

Just make sure to stick to it!

www.facebook.com/healthysmoothierecipes

Smoothies Are Like C

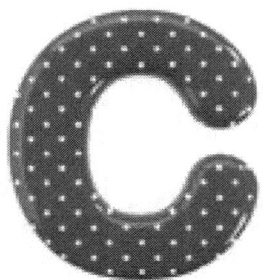

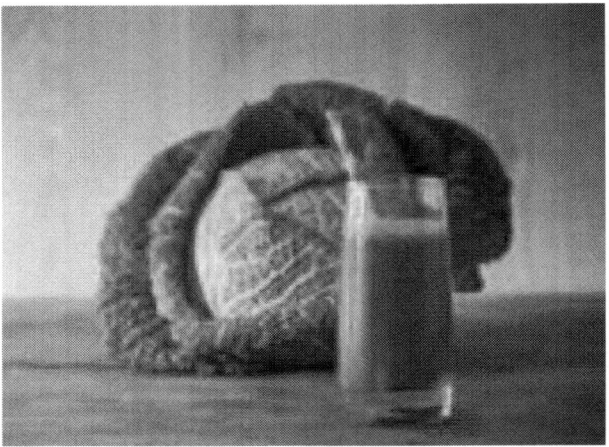

Smoothies are pretty much like the letter C because Smoothies can sometimes be a challenge to balance.
You don't want one that has a challenge with the orange.
Never buy your blender from a public offender because you can not trust such a schlender.
You want to use a quality blender because you want to achieve some kind of relieve.
Never even look at these pretender vendors who only want to sell you fake blenders.

www.facebook.com/healthysmoothiesrecipes

Instead be a big spender and mark your purchase in your calendar because buying a nice quality blender will always render your Smoothie into a tender splendor.

Don't believe me? Let's hear it from Johnny Carson:

Never continue in a job you don't enjoy. If you're happy in what you're doing, you'll like yourself, you'll have inner peace. And if you have that, along with physical health, you will have had more success than you could possibly have imagined. -Johnny Carson

"I'm Going to Make him a Green Smoothie he can't Refuse." -Famous Smoothie Quote

So make sure to stick to the winning Smoothie ingredients that include all the healthy nutrients!

www.facebook.com/healthysmoothierecipes

Smoothies Are Like D

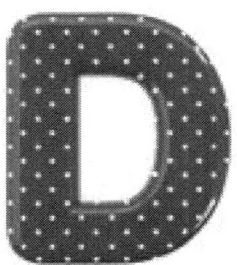

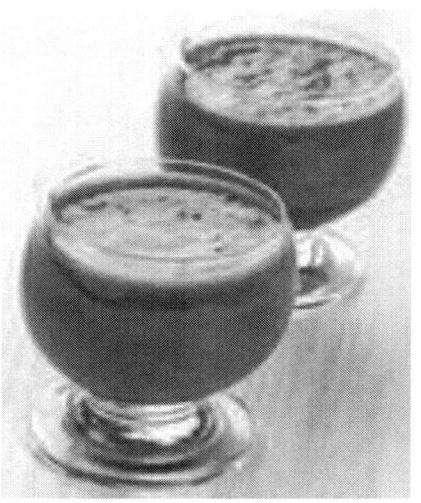

Smoothies are also a lot like the letter D.
Smoothies can help you detox lots and lots.
This is good for you because like this you do not have to run in your reeboks because this Smoothie exercise of detox is better than any exercise of Yoga called peacock.
To summarize go ahead and accessorize yourself with your free enterprise called The Smoothie Lifestyle.
Smoothies are just the best way to energize and to memorize. They are just the new way of aerobic exercise because let me tell you this.

www.facebook.com/healthysmoothiesrecipes

The Smoothie detox is better than bagles and lox.

If you stick to eating your desserts without any grains and flours and dairy, you won't get sick!

Dont't believe me let's hear it from Darwin.

"It is not the strongest of the species that survives, nor the most intelligent that survives. It is the one that is the most adaptable to change." -Darwin

"Green Smoothie, I think this is the Beginning of a Beautiful Relationship." -Famous Smoothie Quote

Adapt your drinks to the Smoothie ratio and you will double your life.

Yes, double and quite the opposite of trouble!

www.facebook.com/healthysmoothierecipes

Smoothies Are Like E

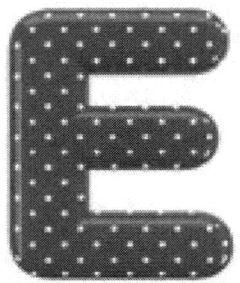

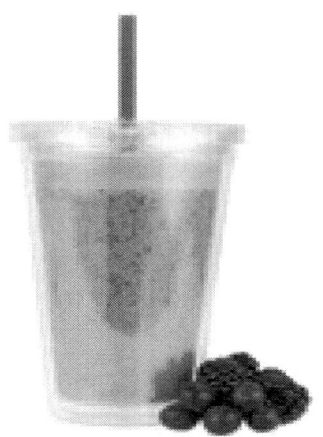

Smoothies are much like the letter E because Smoothies are great for energy.
They are also very good for an allergy because Smoothie veggies cleverly energize you every day.
Energy is good for your memory and potentially you can beat any lethargy with the right smoothie synergy.
To keep your energy flow on the go you might delight Joe from the Smoothie-Chateau.

www.facebook.com/healthysmoothiesrecipes

Should you ever buy your smoothie on the go from the Smoothie-Chateau always make sure to close the lid and always drink slow.

If you do not apply that power grid and close that lid or if you are overexposing somebody might just dispose their nose into your purple scrumptiousness which is of course not the purpose of this so you better drink slow and on your toe.

If you think biodiversity is not worth it, let me tell you, stick to alkaline earth food and you will never get sick!

Here is what Elizabeth Harrison has to say to this:

"Those who are lifting the world upward and onward are those who encourage more than criticize." -Elizabeth Harrison

Always be uplifting, cheerful and be eating wonderful Smoothie ingredient minerals and you can say goodbye to your own funeral!

www.facebook.com/healthysmoothierecipes

Smoothies Are Like F

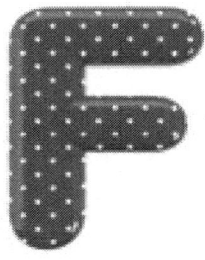

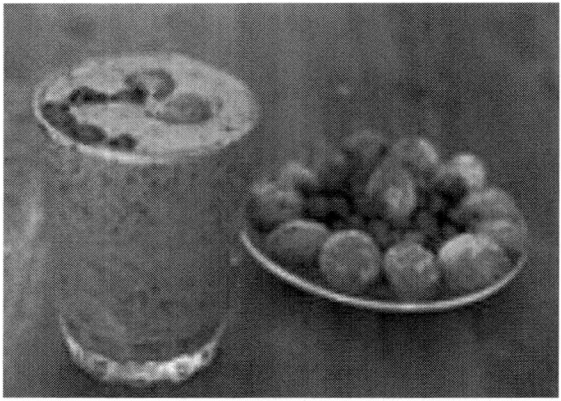

Smoothies remind me a lot of the letter F because Smoothies can be tasty with frozen berries.
Whenever you'd like to enjoy a smoothie don't worry you don't even have to fly to the Canaries to pick fresh berries.
You can buy your berries like frozen cherries and you do not even have to go to Paris.
So go ahead and cherish your berries once a day and I promise your health will never be risqué because smoothies keep the decay away.
Didn't you know Smoothies are a miracle play!

If you do not think cake tasting Smoothies or shakes are important Paleo ingredients get this:

www.facebook.com/healthysmoothiesrecipes

"A Green Smoothie is Worth a Thousand Donuts" -Famous Smoothie Quote

www.facebook.com/healthysmoothierecipes

Smoothies Are Like G

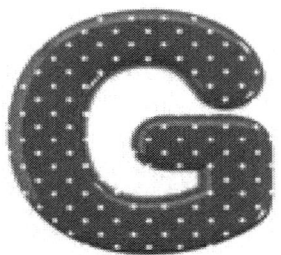

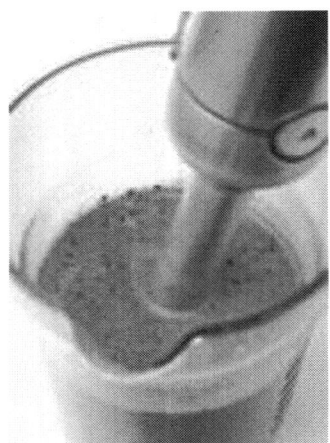

Smoothies are just like the letter G because Smoothies are for good health, yes sometimes they can even bring you great wealth.
Most certainly a scrumptious smoothie is going to take your breath away because it is even better than the best parfait, souflé and sorbet.
A smoothie a day will most certainly be healthier than a peanut butter chocolate bar because with a smoothie in your hand you are the one who is going to the promised land.

www.facebook.com/healthysmoothiesrecipes

Just drink a smoothie every day and you can say bye-bye to that greasy porky pie and everything fried.
With a smoothie a day you are the blazing star not the peanut butter bar.
Heck, who needs a candy bar when a healthy Smoothie is really much more dandy.
Leave the common candy alone and join the Smoothie combat zone because Smoothies build up your muscle tone.
Didn't you notice?
The world needs a serious smoothie zone and not another sugar addicted pudding clone!

If you don't believe me, you might get a reality check here:

"First they ignore you, then they laugh at you, then they fight you, then you win." -Gandhi

www.facebook.com/healthysmoothierecipes

Smoothies Are Like H

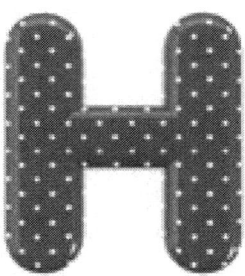

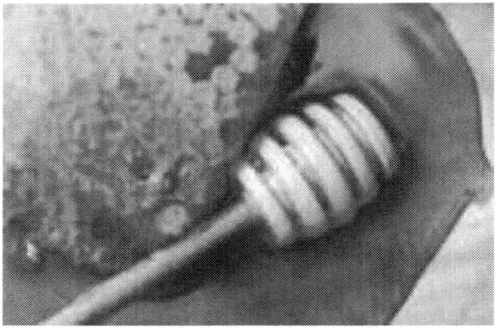

Smoothies are a lot like the letter H because Smoothies can even be enjoyed with some pure organic honey.
Always make sure to secure the pure and never buy the obscure because not only is it immature, but worse it does not even cure.
Honey is really comparable to haute couture and only the mature green manure reassures the honey is pure.
This is the only sureness to test the pureness because pure honey is the only honey that is good for your chest and the only one that your body will
digest without detest.
So the next time when you invest make sure to protest if some possessed pest or someone from the wild west wants to sell

www.facebook.com/healthysmoothiesrecipes

honey with un-pure properties because if you do your body might get infested and congested.

Never buy honey from someone who got arrested and never buy from someone who is untested!

Let me tell you this. If you stick to it, you will never get sick!

Leigh Hunt can really speak to this:

The groundwork of all happiness is health. -Leigh Hunt

Just make sure to stick to it!

Smoothies Are Like I

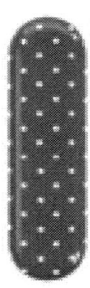

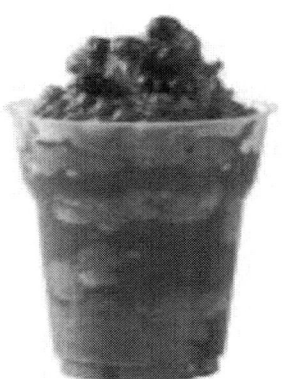

Smoothies are just a lot like the letter I because ice cream smoothies put everyone's esteem upstream.
You might think that ice cream smoothies are only good with whipping cream, but whipping and dipping are not the kind of nipping if fitting in your clothes is the pose you chose!
You can redeem a serious regime with a healthy Smoothie routine.
The American dream might look like strawberry ice cream, but do you really want to be part of the heavy beam team?
Well, if you want to show your seriousness and get straight with your ice cream smoothie due date because you want to fight that weight make sure to only use LITE.

www.facebook.com/healthysmoothiesrecipes

Take in the serious minerals and keep out the heavy cereal.
I told you. The ice cream smoothie diet only works in a way that is lite.
Your dream does not consist of any sort of cream because your reality of supreme looks like the organic and pure Smoothie cuisine:

Lean & Clean!

Let me tell you this. If you stick to it, you will never get sick!

Ivan Illich can really speak to this:

Healthy people are those who live in healthy homes on a healthy diet; in an environment equally fit for birth, growth work, healing, and dying... Healthy people need no bureaucratic interference to mate, give birth, share the human condition and die. -Ivan Illich

Just make sure to stick to it!

www.facebook.com/healthysmoothierecipes

Smoothies Are Like J

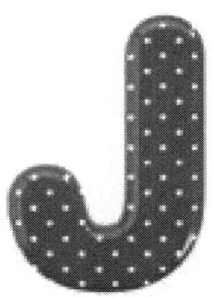

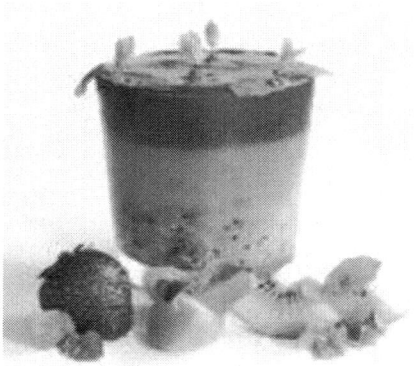

Smoothies are just like the letter J because Smoothies are better than juicing can ever be.
That's because you get more nutrients from smoothies, you see, so make sure to go on that healthy smoothie ingredients shopping spree.
The health nuts all agree.
Pure black tea is not good for your health, but on the other hand, smoothies balanced out with a mix of green peas, black tea, hembree, herb tea, fruit tea and yuichi are key.
You see smoothies offer lots of possibilities and you can even drink them with ghee.

www.facebook.com/healthysmoothiesrecipes

So, let's say yippee and ye-yi to planting our own banana tree because in our Smoothies we need lots of Vitamin C.

Let me tell you this. If you stick to it, you will never get sick!

John Wooden can really speak to a situation like this:

"Perfection is impossible. However striving for perfection is not. Do the best you can under the conditions that exist. That is what counts." -John Wooden

www.facebook.com/healthysmoothierecipes

Smoothies Are Like K

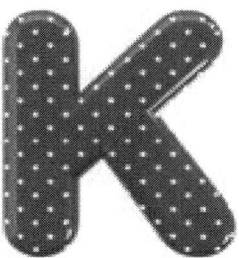

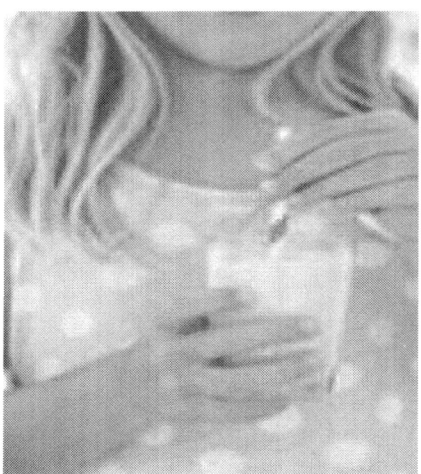

Smoothies are like the letter K because Smoothies are fun for kids to drink in pink plus they provide a good source of zinc. Kids do not only love mini smoothies that are great to take for a snack in their backpack, but all children agree that drinking smoothies with a lot of zinc is even more fun if the smoothies are in colors like Indian pink, Japanese pink and yellowish pink.

Here is a very wise man who can speak to this and I assure you this will give you the kicks:

www.facebook.com/healthysmoothiesrecipes

"Most people work hard and spend their health trying to achieve wealth. Then they retire and spend their wealth trying to get back their health." -Kevin Gianni

www.facebook.com/healthysmoothierecipes

Smoothies Are Like L

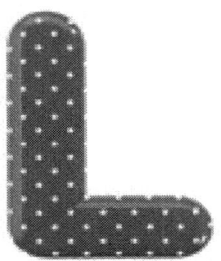

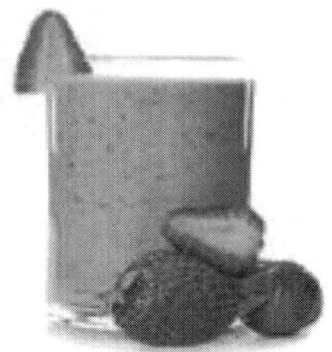

Smoothies remind me of the letter L because Smoothies make life quite wonderful, yes they make life grand.
Yet on the other hand, make sure to develop your whip hand if you are not a big spender in case you do not want to buy that blender.
Smoothies are great for young and old and no matter if you are whipping your smoothies with a flipping mixing ninja or if you understand how to whip by hand.
In any case and no matter what brand or how you expand, Smoothies are going to take you to that Promised Land!

www.facebook.com/healthysmoothiesrecipes

On the other hand, Loving Mother Teresa knows exactly what it is:

"Love is a fruit in season at all times, and within the reach of every hand." - Mother Teresa

www.facebook.com/healthysmoothierecipes

Smoothies Are Like M

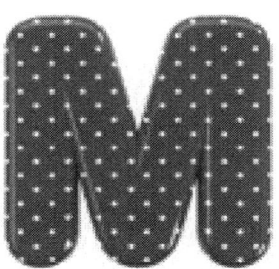

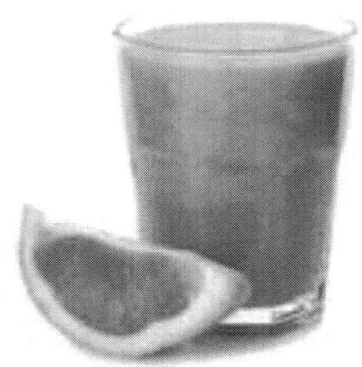

Smoothies have an awful lot in common with the letter M.
Smoothies are great for mindfulness and they can keep you really sharp.
Did you know that Smoothies are even healthier than eating carp because with Smoothies there is no cheating.
If you want to maintain a sharp memory make sure to think about the following concern.
You only want to turn ingredients like cinnamon fern, aspargus fern and licorice fern.

www.facebook.com/healthysmoothiesrecipes

Once you decide to become healthy there is no point of return. Postpone your appointment with Joan because your muscle tone is more important than watching that film of Sierra Leone.

Let me tell you this. If you stick to it, you will never get sick!

Marc Aurelius can really speak to this because he has the experience:

"The wise man sees in the misfortune of others what he should avoid." -Marcus Aurelius

www.facebook.com/healthysmoothierecipes

Smoothies Are Like N

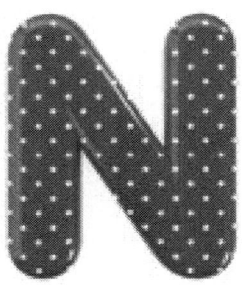

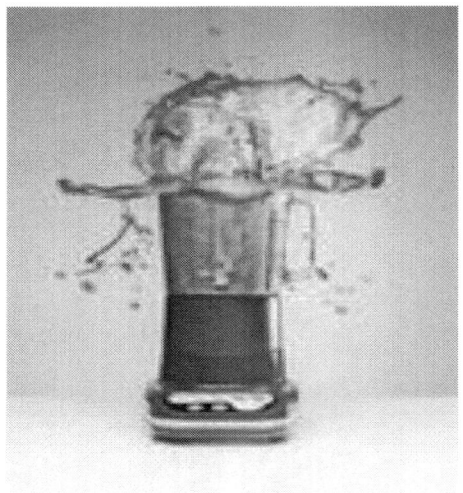

Smoothies truly remind me of the letter N.
Smoothies with a Nutribullet also make your treatment conveniently fast.
Remember your Smoothie achievement is not only ingenious, but it is totally convenient because if you are obedient and follow the right ingredients
you will not only be fast, but you will be considered unsurpassed!

www.facebook.com/healthysmoothiesrecipes

So make sure to drink one every day to maintain a full tummy feeling that is really revealing and provides you with that ultimate healing.

Let me tell you this. If you stick to it, you will never get sick!

Niccolo Machiavelli can really speak to this:

Develop the strength to do bold things, not the strength to suffer. -Niccolo Machiavelli, The Prince

Just make sure to stick to it!

www.facebook.com/healthysmoothierecipes

Smoothies Are Like O

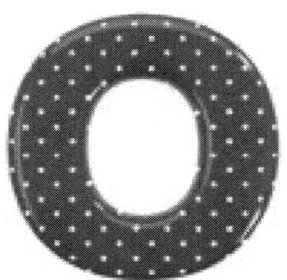

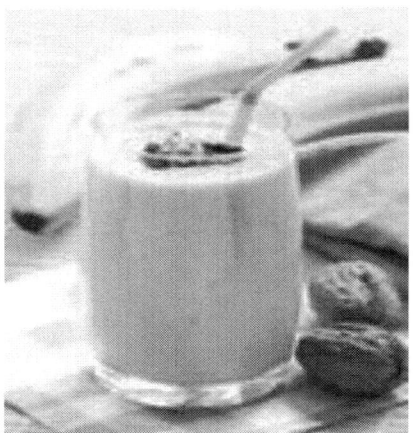

Smoothies are really much like the letter O.
Smoothies that are organic can provide some chemical-free good stuff.
If you don't care about chemical-free stuff and think the issue with Smoothies is polemical, you should consider the following miracle.
Eating and drinking chemical-free stuff is not only ethical, but the people who work in the medical obstacle say chemical-free makes you more flexible and on the physical level it makes you even more sensual.

www.facebook.com/healthysmoothiesrecipes

Drinking chemical-free smoothies provides you with a typical vegetal festival says the health professional staff.
So make sure to blend them up just right and you'll get lots of healthy smoothie fluff!

It is true Smoothie lovers go against the grain which is an outlook that is shared by Oscar Wilde, too:

"Everything that is popular is wrong." -Oscar Wilde

"We Are such Stuff As Green Smoothies are Made of..." - Famous Smoothie Quote

www.facebook.com/healthysmoothierecipes

Smoothies Are Like P

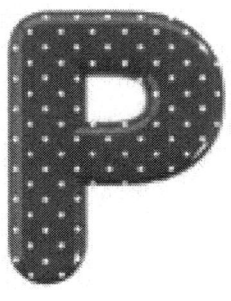

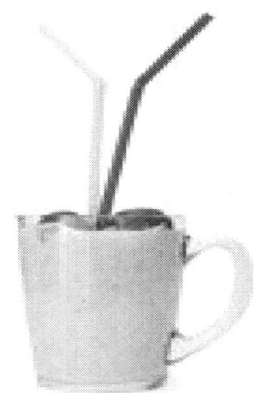

Smoothies are much like the letter P.
Smoothies can help develop perfect pink skin that doesn't flake, break or ache.
On the other hand, the skin of folks who have a ton of sponge and pound cake breaks always flakes.
For god's sake make sure to drop that cake and replace it with the healthy shake.
Better yet, if you can't drop the cake, go ahead and use the shake that tastes like cake.

www.facebook.com/healthysmoothiesrecipes

If you can't get rid of these nasty potato chips, you might try a miracle dip.

Sipping that dip will make you smart as whip and without going on that nasty guilt trip because with Smoothies you can still enjoy the taste of

chips, but you can stay on your pleasure trips.

Smoothies can really taste rich and just like your favorite tortilla chip.

I hope you get the pic.

Smoothies are healthier than chips because with Smoothies you get more water with every single sip!

Let me tell you this. If you stick to Smoothies, you will never get sick!

Peter Pitrelli can really attest to this:

"True silence is the rest of the mind, and is to the spirit what sleep is to the body, nourishment and refreshment." - William Penn

Just make sure to stick to it!

www.facebook.com/healthysmoothierecipes

Smoothies Are Like Q

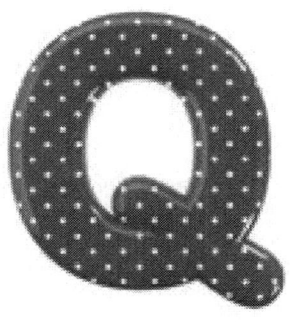

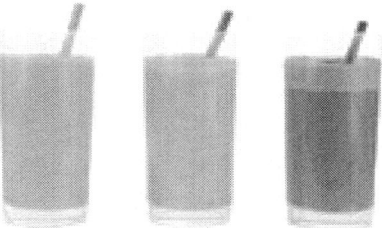

Smoothies are making me think of the letter Q.
Smoothies made with quinoa can give you more fiber than you'll know.
The cold and hard hitting truth is just like this.
Smoothies, you know, are desired by those who are called survivors.
Survivors are flexible and agile and pretty quick much like Bengal tigers, spiders, or vipers and quite the opposite of candy stripers.
Smoothie survivors are pretty rough riders because they are providers of potential dividers.
These survivors are are also quite the opposite of alcoholic cider passionates.

www.facebook.com/healthysmoothiesrecipes

Smoothie fans are compassionate devil's advocates of miraculous and fabulous nutritious happiness.

Yes, Smoothie lovers are rebels and they are insiders who know how to build up internal muscle fibers.

Let me tell you this. If you stick to it, you will never get sick!

Quincy Hawthorne can really speak to this:

"The only exercise some people get is jumping to conclusions, running down their friends, side-stepping their responsibilities, and pushing their luck!" -Quincy Hawthorne

Just make sure to stick to it!

www.facebook.com/healthysmoothierecipes

Smoothies Are Like R

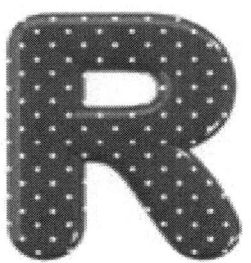

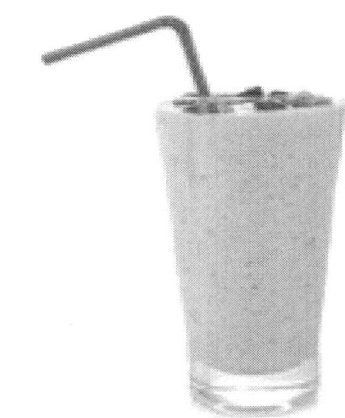

Smoothies have a lot in common with the letter R.
Smoothies are great for runners because they give an energy groove.
Runners who drink Smoothies do not only feel the groove, but they are certainly runners who are improved.
Smoothies can help a runner's feet because Smoothie runners are the elite that beat the wheat.
Smoothie runners defeat everyone else and without having to retreat to reading vanity fair to keep their sanity.
Smoothie runners also apply reasonable care because their affair is taking the time that they can spare and tear through

beet root, bamboo shoot, sweet fruit in order to make the most scrumptious banana passion fruit pursuit.

Let me tell you this. If you stick to it, you will never get sick!

Richard Branson can really speak to this:

As an adventurer...I try to protect against the downside. I make sure I have covered as many eventualities as I can. In the end, you have to take calculated risks; otherwise you're going to sit in mothballs all day and do nothing. -Richard Branson

Just make sure to stick to it!

www.facebook.com/healthysmoothierecipes

Smoothies Are Like S

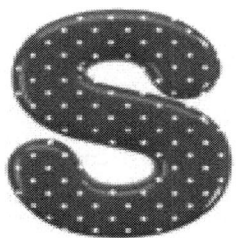

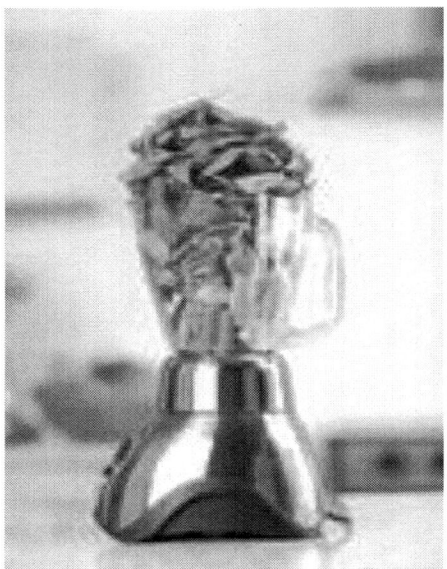

Smoothies are always reminding me of the letter S because Smoothies made with spinach can quickly add to your health in a very swift way.
On one hand, this is good for your intake of vitamin K and on the other hand Smoothies are good to cast away that nasty radioactive decay.
They also uplift your spiritual bouquet and they are a great way to turn away from pancake day.

www.facebook.com/healthysmoothiesrecipes

Let me tell you this. If you stick to it, you will never get sick! Satchel Paige can really speak to this because she knows this technique:

"The time to relax is when you don't have time for it." - Satchel Paige

Just make sure to stick to it!

Smoothies Are Like T

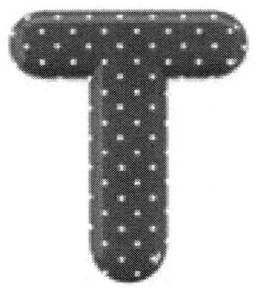

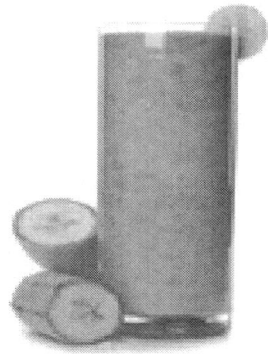

Smoothies are really a lot like the letter T.
Smoothies are great for your thyroid because drinking it can help you regulate.
Smoothies stimulate and regenerate your esprit de corps and your mental score.
Never underestimate your endeavor because if you are drinking Smoothies you will live forever.

Let me tell you this. If you stick to it, you will never get sick!

www.facebook.com/healthysmoothiesrecipes

The 14th Dalai Lama can also speak to this because he knows his technique:

**"Remember that silence is sometimes the best answer."
~Tenzin Gyatso, the 14th Dalai Lama**

Just make sure to stick to it!

www.facebook.com/healthysmoothierecipes

Smoothies Are Like U

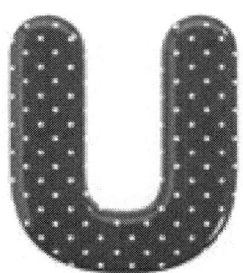

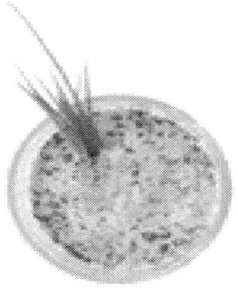

Smoothies remind me a lot of the letter U because Smoothies under 100 calories are filling the body's batteries in an incredibly fulfilling way.
You'll soon be addicted to them because they're quite wonderful!
The reason why Smoothies are so addictive is the fact that they are truly unrestricted.
Yes, Smoothies are not only wonderful, but you can enjoy these powerful minerals plentiful.

And as always, never, never forget this.

If you stick to it, you will never get sick!

Umberto Ungerer can really speak to this:

"The only exercise some people get is jumping to conclusions, running down their friends, side-stepping their responsibilities, and pushing their luck!" -Umberto Ungerer

"I love the smell of Green Smoothies in the morning. It Smells like Victory!" -Famous Smoothie Quote

So, please make sure to stick to it!

www.facebook.com/healthysmoothierecipes

Smoothies Are Like V

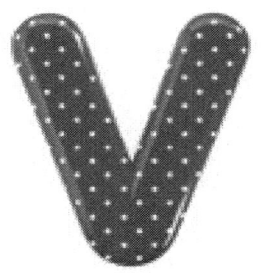

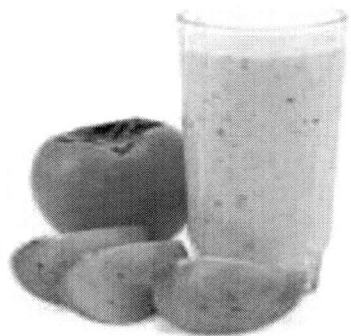

Smoothies are really a lot like the letter V.
Smoothies made with a Vitamix can be done in less than five minutes and that is what I call a quick fix.
There are plenty of tricks to make a Smoothie even a quicker fix.
This bag of tricks is always giving me the kicks when I mix.
A cranberry elixir and a peach twister taste so sweet without the unhealthy wheat and did you know that such a nutritious twister can even heal your fever blister?
Yes, these Smoothies are powerful and perfect for folks who need nutrition for their ignition and condition because that is how they beat their competition.

www.facebook.com/healthysmoothiesrecipes

The best ingredients you can use are bamboo shoot, citrus fruit, kiwi fruit, pepper fruit, blueberry root, celery root and horseradish root.

Let me tell you this. If you stick to it, you will never get sick!

Virgil can also speak to this:

"They can because they think they can." -Virgil

"Are you Telling Me you Built a Time Machine… out of a Vita-Mix?" -Famous Smoothie Quote

Just make sure to stick to it!

www.facebook.com/healthysmoothierecipes

Smoothies Are Like W

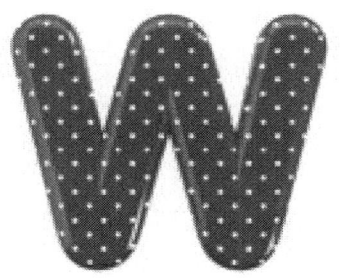

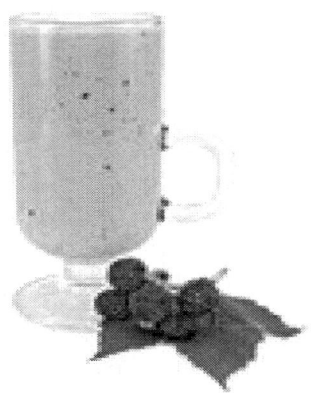

Smoothies are an awful lot like the letter W because Smoothies made with winter fruit can be wonderful and flavorful until you refill and take your power drill.
Smoothies also help a lot to energize and they are good for your exercise.
A melon elixir made with a mixer is a mixture that is richer and thicker than malt liquor.
In addition it gives you a bigger kicker than any pot liquor.

www.facebook.com/healthysmoothiesrecipes

Always remember that Smoothies unlike alcohol are the heavier hitters because Smoothies are serious spark transmitters. Not only are Smoothies designated hitters, but Smoothies are giving you the vigor and when you pull that blender trigger Smoothies are just bigger than any juice abuse!

Let me tell you this. If you stick to it, you will never get sick!

Winston Churchill can also speak to this because he knows the technique:

"When you're going through hell, keep going." -Winston Churchill

"Now is the Winter of our Green Smoothies" -Famous Smoothie Quote

www.facebook.com/healthysmoothierecipes

Smoothies Are Like X

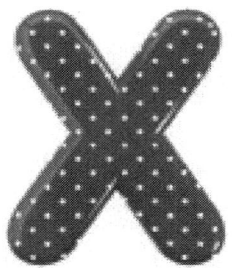

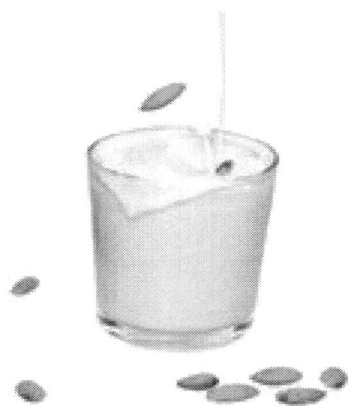

Smoothies remind me a lot of the letter X because a Smoothie xchange is forever.
Smoothies are also great because they help you kill that excessive weight.
They are also good for your heart rate and typically when you enjoy them late you will always find a soul mate who will give you the latest Smoothie updates telling you about the perfect ingredient dose rates.

www.facebook.com/healthysmoothiesrecipes

At any rate, Smoothie soul mates are great because now you got yourself a new running mate to help you lose that nasty body weight.

Let me tell you this. If you stick to it, you will never get sick!

Xao Oz can also speak to this because he knows the technique:

"Nobody can go back and start a new beginning, but anyone can start today and make a new ending." -Xao Oz

www.facebook.com/healthysmoothierecipes

Smoothies Are Like Y

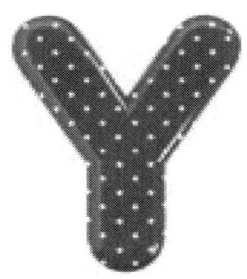

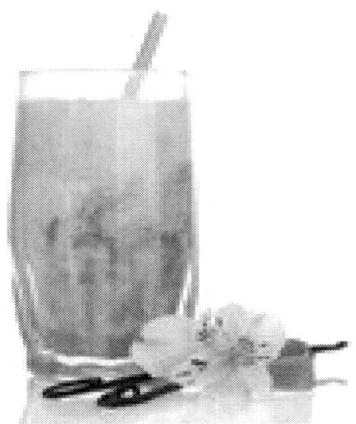

Smoothies are a lot like the letter Y because ultimately Smoothies are keeping you in connection with your Yin & Yang and 24/7.
When you drink one every day you'll crank it up to eleven!
Once you are in the Ying & Yang zone you will be able to climb on that famous Smoothie throne.
You also want to notice that with Smoothies you will never have to worry about your hip bone or your kidney stone.

www.facebook.com/healthysmoothiesrecipes

With a tight muscle tone you will never have to buy a participation loan because your bone is now as valuable as precious stone.

Once you are in the Yin & Yang zone you do not need a stepping stone loan to insure your allure.

I hope by now you can see why Smoothies are related to Ying & Yang and the number seven because, my friends, smoothies are just sent from heaven.

To sum it up in a few words:

The Smoothie diet is the way to go because it will bring you the avid habit of eternity and with Smoothies you will live the life of biodiversity, harmony and sanity!

Smoothies, my friend, are the elixir of life.

I hope by now you get my point of view because **Smoothies are just like You!**

Let me tell you this. If you stick to it, you will never get sick!

Martin Yan can also speak to this because he knows the technique:

"People who don't travel cannot have a global view, all they see is what's in front of them. Those people cannot accept new things because all they know is where they live." - Martin Yan

www.facebook.com/healthysmoothierecipes

Smoothies Are Like Z

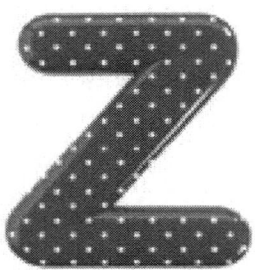

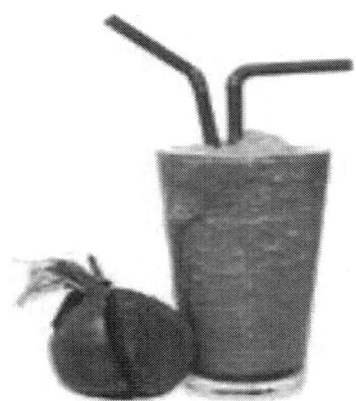

Smoothies are just like the letter Z because Smoothies are keeping you in the zone.
Smoothies are also great because they're so easy to make. Why not try one for yourself right now for goodness sake!
From apples to bananas, oranges to strawberries, and everything in between, with a smoothie every day your health goals can be met faster than anyone has ever seen!
With Smoothies you want to focus on green beans to make your system clean.
Smoothies offer a lot of variety, too.

www.facebook.com/healthysmoothiesrecipes

If you want to live a healthy smoothie lifestyle, you do not even need to be part of the high society because all you need is some creativity, selectivity and productivity.

With Smoothies you can also lose that nasty weight and you will soon feel like Alexander The Great with an even better metabolic rate.

With Smoothies you do not even have to infuse because you can amuse yourself with ingredients like aspargus bean in dandelion green, vanilla bean, tangerine, potato bean in olive green, soya bean and sage green sardine.

You can use berries like cherries and these are better than drinking caffeine to push your adrenaline.

Smoothies are the true golden mean and whenever you feel unclean make sure to go on that supervisory green routine called the **Green Smoothie Regime.**

Let me tell you this. If you stick to it, you will never get sick!

Here is yet another quick kick:

"Be not afraid of growing slowly, be afraid only of standing still." ~Chinese Proverb

"May the Smoothie be with you...Always" -Famous Smoothie Quote

And always, always remember stick to it because

Smoothies Are Like You!

www.facebook.com/healthysmoothierecipes

Conclusion

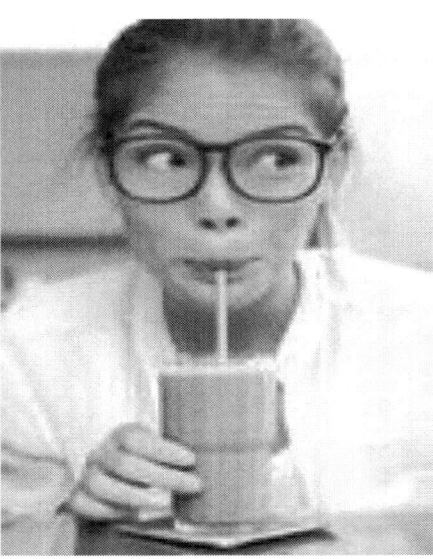

Smoothies every day can help you change your life.
It can be the tool that is needed to eliminate your life's strife.
A few minutes is all it takes to explore and find an answer to how Smoothie lovers are drinking lean and clean instead of running to that butter cream dream.
Clean is a Smoothie lover's theme and you will find that practicing the law of the Smoothie lifestyle is guaranteed to bring to you that world view of true and organic grew bamboo pursue, too, because the Smoothie law is tried and true and with Smoothies you'll never catch that nasty stomach flu!

"All Great Things are Simple, and Many can be Expressed in Single Words: Freedom, Justice, Honor, Duty, Mercy, Hope, Smoothies." -Famous Smoothies

www.facebook.com/healthysmoothiesrecipes

More Scrumptiousness

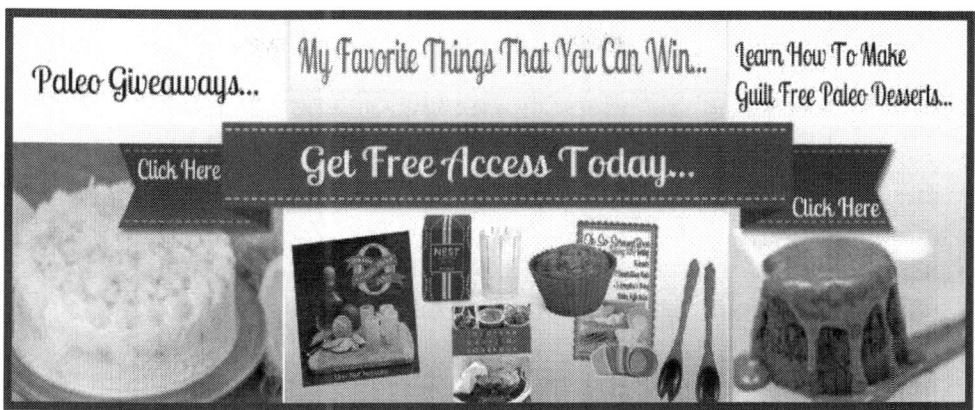

To get access to The Unforgettable Paleo Moments where you will get even more Paleo lifestyle pleasures, including some magical "Oprah" Paleo Favorite Things and other delightful guilt free Paleo goodies that will help you with your own Paleo experience in a big way, check out the link below...

More Smoothie Paleo Moments...Unforgettable Smoothie Pleasures: http://ohmyfavoritethings.com

About The Author

Juliana Baldec lives the Paleo lifestyle and the Smoothie lifestyle herself. She is also a very passionate health author and publisher and has written several book series about the Smoothie Lifestyle and the Paleo Smoothie lifestyle as well as Fast Juicing and a series of Health Recipes for Life and a series of yoga and meditation books.

Her story of recovery from an incurable illness has inspired her over the years to help many other sufferers around the world. She has found a cure of her Asthma and sleeping problem by sticking to a Smoothie or better yet Paleo Smoothie lifestyle.

People remember her because she changes their lives with scrumptious recipes that provide them with some powerful health befits. She is also known for making a healthy smoothie diet or better yet a healthy smoothie lifestyle achievable and realistic for regular people who are not able to spend a lot of money for expensive ingredients or who do not have a lot of time because they are busy.

She gives them a real solution for their busy lifestyles.

Juliana was born and raised in Memphis where she spent most of her life growing up in the beautiful country side.

The country not only taught her how to appreciate natural foods, but also how to appreciate the use of fresh, organic and gluten free ingredients in her cooking and lifestyle.

Her love for what the country had to offer quickly turned into her passion for cooking with a purpose. Each food and each ingredient is a gift of good and helps heal, cleanse, energize, or benefit the body in some specific way.

www.facebook.com/healthysmoothiesrecipes

Being able to assemble the knowledge about foods and ingredients that are beneficial for the body and brain has enabled her to heal her own illness even though she has been discouraged by her doctors who told her that her illness was incurable.

Based on her own results and the results of her clients, Juliana loves to teach other people how to cook the healthy way, how to follow a healthy and happy lifestyle by using the proper ingredients and she loves achieving results for her clients based on applying the proper ingredients and foods.

In order to share and put out her message that the proper ingredients and food have the power to heal the body, Juliana decided to start writing her own books on cooking, dieting, juicing, the smoothie lifestyle, the Paleo lifestyle, yoga, meditation and many other health related topics that involve the proper foods and ingredients. Showing people how to get achievable and realistic results with these ingredients is her main focus.

She likes to use affordable means without sacrificing the quality so that everybody has the chance to change sick making habits into an affordable and healthy lifestyle with amazing results that everyone who respects the rules can achieve in a quick and easy way and even if one thinks he or she is too busy.

www.facebook.com/healthysmoothierecipes

More Information

If you enjoy my work, please feel free to join our facebook pages at:

http://www.facebook.com/healthysmoothiesrecipes

And if you are interested in learning more about our other products and publications, please visit:

Juliana Baldec's Books:

Go to Google, Goodreads or your favorite online marketplace and type the author name "Juliana Baldec" into the search box to find all her book series and upcoming new book releases.

More Smoothie Scrumptiousness:

http://www.facebook.com/healthysmoothiesrecipes

Unforgettable Smoothie Pleasures
http://ohmyfavoritethings.com

More Paleo Moments

Unforgettable Smoothie Pleasures
http://ohmyfavoritethings.com

www.facebook.com/healthysmoothiesrecipes

www.facebook.com/healthysmoothierecipes

www.facebook.com/healthysmoothiesrecipes

www.facebook.com/healthysmoothierecipes

Made in the USA
Middletown, DE
09 April 2017